HEAL YOURSELF HEAL THE WORLD

DEBORAH KING

ATRIA PAPERBACK
New York London Toronto Sydney New Delhi

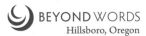 BEYOND WORDS
Hillsboro, Oregon

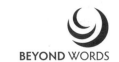

BEYOND WORDS

A Division of Simon & Schuster, Inc.
1230 Avenue of the Americas
New York, NY 10020

20827 N.W. Cornell Road, Suite 500
Hillsboro, Oregon 97124-9808
503-531-8700 / 503-531-8773 fax
www.beyondword.com

This publication contains the opinions and ideas of its author. It is intended to provide helpful and informative material on the subjects addressed in the publication. It is sold with the understanding that the author and publisher are not engaged in rendering medical, health, or any other kind of personal professional services in the book. The reader should consult his or her medical, health, or other competent professional before adopting any of the suggestions in this book or drawing inferences from it. The author and publisher specifically disclaim all responsibility for any liability, loss or risk, personal or otherwise, which is incurred as a consequence, directly or indirectly, of the use and application of any of the contents of this book.

Managing editor: Lindsay S. Easterbrooks-Brown
Editor: Sarah Heilman
Copyeditor: Ali Shaw
Proofreader: Linda M. Meyer
Artwork: Alice Charlier
Cover design: Sara E. Blum
Composition: William H. Brunson Typography Services

First Atria Paperback/Beyond Words trade paperback edition October 2017

ATRIA PAPERBACK, logo, and colophon are trademarks of Simon & Schuster, Inc.
BEYOND WORDS PUBLISHING, logo, and colophon are registered trademarks of Beyond Words Publishing. Beyond Words is an imprint of Simon & Schuster, Inc.

For more information about special discounts for bulk purchases, please contact Simon & Schuster Special Sales at 1-866-506-1949 or business@simonandschuster.com.

The Simon & Schuster Speakers Bureau can bring authors to your live event. For more information or to book an event, contact the Simon & Schuster Speakers Bureau at 1-866-248-3049 or visit our website at www.simonspeakers.com.

Manufactured in the United States of America

10 9 8 7 6 5 4 3 2

Library of Congress Cataloging-in-Publication Data:
Names: King, Deborah, author.
Title: Heal yourself—heal the world / Deborah King.
Description: First Atria Paperback/Beyond Words trade paperback edition. |
 New York : Atria Paperback ; Hillsboro, Oregon : Beyond Words, 2017. |
Identifiers: LCCN 2017003896 (print) | LCCN 2017013240 (ebook) |
 ISBN 9781501132063 (eBook) | ISBN 9781582705866 (paperback)
Subjects: LCSH: Energy medicine. | Healing. | Mind and body therapies. |
 Self-care, Health. | BISAC: BODY, MIND & SPIRIT / Healing / General. |
 HEALTH & FITNESS / Healthy Living. | SELF-HELP / Personal Growth / Happiness. |
Classification: LCC RZ421 (ebook) | LCC RZ421 .K56 2017 (print) |
 DDC 615.8/52—dc23
LC record available at https://lccn.loc.gov/2017003896

The corporate mission of Beyond Words Publishing, Inc.: *Inspire to Integrity*

Dedication

To Eric—my husband, my best friend, my spiritual partner . . . always.

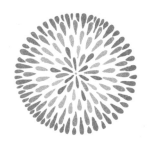

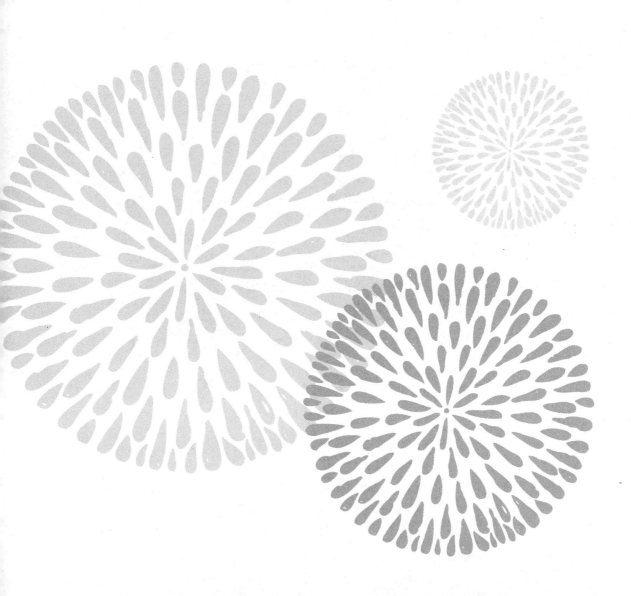

CONTENTS

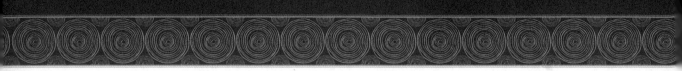

Part III: Using Your Power to Heal Others

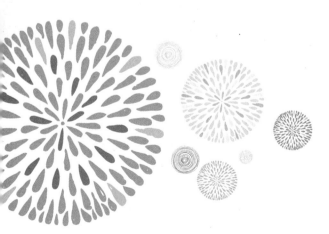

FOREWORD

'm an electrical engineering and computer science graduate. A classic geek who reads science books for fun and entertainment. As such, much of what Deborah teaches should be dismissed by my rational, scientific mind. Energy healing should be nothing more than outdated beliefs from shamanic or ancient practices that existed long before the silicon age.

Except that I can't.

Over the last three decades, I've had experiences with energy healing that defy explanation. No matter how I tried, my scientific mind could not explain them. My doctors attributed them to the placebo effect, which is nothing more than simply saying, "It worked. We don't know how, but your mind did it."

This is why I feel Deborah's work is so important. While we cannot scientifically explain how energy healing works, we know that it does. And for many people, it goes beyond just physical healing into healing one's emotional state, feelings about the world, and self-esteem. It's inexplicable but powerful stuff.

I like to explain it to my fellow left-brained minds as follows: For thousands of years mankind has used the sun for multiple purposes—from navigation, to providing warmth and light, to growing crops, to telling time. Yet it's only been in the last one hundred years that we finally figured out how the sun worked—a giant thermonuclear reaction made up of hydrogen and helium atoms.

But not knowing how the sun worked—as we've only known this for a tiny slice of humanity's time on earth—didn't prevent our forefathers from using the sun. Perhaps it's the same with energy healing. Someday, a few hundred years from now, we might understand the connections between meridian lines, chakras, auras, and our physical bodies, but right now, not knowing the explanation does not prevent us from using it. Its multiple uses are so magnificent that we don't have to fully understand *how* it works in order to reap its amazing benefits.

I founded MindvalleyAcademy.com in 2013 to bring education of this sort into the mainstream. We seek out pools of knowledge that we know are truly important to healthy, happy human lives but which have not yet been included in mainstream education. Deborah is one of our most gifted teachers, and we're honored to have published some of her online courses. Her programs have proven extremely popular as they help the deep need so many have of connecting to Spirit and healing from the inside out.

Now Deborah has written this exciting workbook on energy healing, which sets the stage for readers to embrace their inner healer and eventually to be part of the growing wave of consciousness that aims to heal not only ourselves but also the planet. This is the type of education that I applaud: going from personal development and extending outward to lift humanity to higher reaches of awareness and love. Tomorrow's entrepreneurs, tech innovators, philanthropists, educators, and healers will be able to stand tall in the wisdom that brings together the mind, body, and spirit in a healthy, balanced whole.

Heal Yourself—Heal the World takes you on an energy adventure that illuminates the process of embracing your energy—understanding how it shifts and expresses itself through the chakras—and shows you that you really do have the power to heal. Filled with meditations and profound techniques, it's a do-it-yourself guide to healing yourself and to sharing your newfound skills with others, including your pets. Along the way, you'll meet your spiritual guides, learn about meditation and mind/body types (a handy tool indeed), and understand how to stay healthy and in love with your life.

I know you will come to appreciate, as I have, Deborah's deep devotion to healing the planet and its individuals. It's up to all of us to shift our awareness to higher levels and to embrace the inclusiveness and unconditional love that is contained in this book. Now dive in!

Vishen Lakhiani

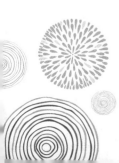

INTRODUCTION

I was not yet twenty-five years old, was just out of law school, and was on the corporate fast track. I was an athlete, participating in extreme sports. And I modeled in size 2s. Despite all these outward signs of success, deep down inside I knew something was very wrong. I was seriously unhappy and out of balance, but I tried not to think about why. Life was busy, and if I ran fast enough or drank enough or popped enough pills, I could keep moving.

Then I was diagnosed with cancer. Talk about a wake-up call!

As I tried to figure out the reasons behind my health issues, I found myself struggling with buried traumas and a difficult childhood. Somewhere in the midst of all the questions, the struggles, and the hurts, I discovered something pretty amazing—energy healing. It wasn't something that you could order from Amazon or pick up at the store. It was a whole new world opening up. The more I learned about energy healing, the more I was convinced that it could rid so much of what was wrong with me and that I could heal.

The reality is that we all have this power to heal within us—yes, even you! You, too, are an energy healer. Believe it. Your power to heal is packed with enough punch to aid in mending those nasty wounds from the past and enough magic to spark your healthy and amazing new life.

Once you see how the power of energy healing can change your own life, you begin to realize that you can use this gift for the benefit of others—your family, your friends, even your pets. As you begin assisting others in their healing, you are, in fact, helping to heal the larger world. The more you grow in awareness and the more you grow in love, the greater your power to help heal those around you. I have found this to be true for me, and I know it can be true for you too.

The Time Is *Now*

Embarking upon the path of healing means orienting to a new way of life. Energy healing will radically shift everything you thought you knew about the world. It serves as a catalyst for a chain reaction that starts with you and radiates out, ultimately spreading out to affect the entire universe. Does this sound amazing? It is! Energy healing is a big deal. There is nothing small about it. This is part of your purpose in being here on earth. You are meant to experience a vibrant life through your body, and by choosing to embark on this journey with me, you're taking an important step toward ensuring that the experience will be a positive one.

In reading this book, you will learn how to effect change in your energy field and in your physical body. You will also discover how your physical body—the temple of your soul—is connected to your emotions, psyche, and spirit and how you can raise your vibration to enter higher and more profound states of awareness and health. I will also provide practical and higher-level energy medicine techniques to support you.

In part I, you'll begin to grasp what's standing between you and the life you know you were truly meant to live. As I share my personal story of pain and healing with you, you'll start to get a sense of how denying the pain you've lived through and bottling up your true feelings are holding you back. You'll begin the energetic healing process by learning how to assess and clear out your own emotional debris. You'll develop an understanding about your chakras (energy centers) as you learn about the seven main energy centers in the body, the eighth chakra (the soul star), and those beyond. You'll learn how to use a pendulum so you can actually see the workings of energy in your chakras and experience the universal energy field for yourself. Next, you'll grasp the basics of initiation and how it can help you become more open and more conscious.

In part II, you'll be taught how to cultivate a powerful meditation practice and how to use specialized practices to revitalize your energy field and balance your chakras. And you'll find that you don't have to walk this path alone; your spiritual guides are here to help! You'll learn the system of mind/body types and defense mechanisms that develop when energy is twisted early in life. From there you will move on to identifying sources of negative energy and what you can do to remove them from your life. Practical exercises as well as powerful tools—such as working with the *hara* line—will be provided along the way so that you can practice what you are studying and immediately apply this new information to create the life you have, until now, only dreamed of.

In part III, you will continue to heal yourself deeply while learning to heal your family, friends, and even your pets through a variety of techniques, such as sound healing and chelation, and including my method, LifeForce Energy Healing®, an instantaneous way to effect change. Then you can move on to helping heal the world. In conclusion, I introduce you to the potency of healing circles and how each one of us can help bring about peace on earth.

By the time you are finished with this book, you will know yourself far more intimately, you will have released the impediments to your own health and happiness, and you will know your purpose in being here on earth. You will have learned what it means to take responsibility for your own healing, and you will have experienced the joy and excitement that comes when you step up to the plate of your own best life.

If you are ready to explore this healing energy that resides within your being, follow me to the first chapter. Welcome to your remarkable healing journey.

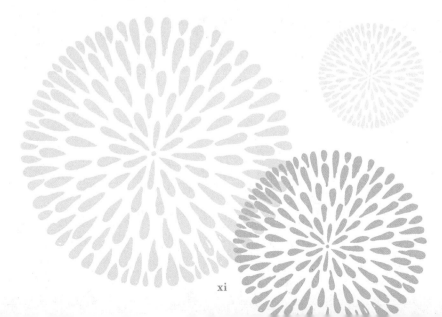

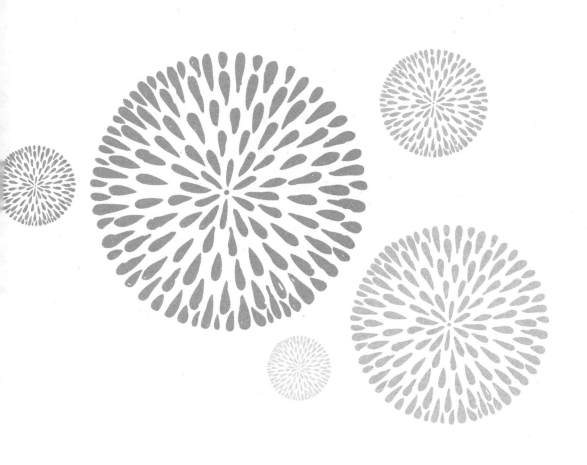

PART I

HOW TO ACTIVATE ENERGY HEALING

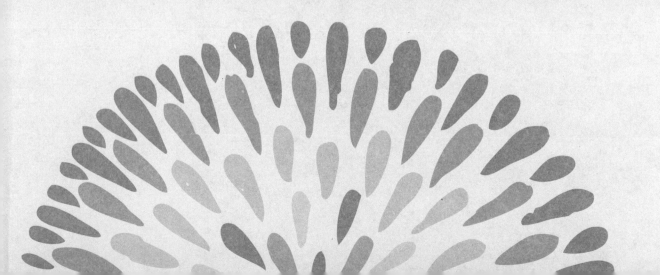

DO I REALLY HAVE THE POWER TO HEAL?

s there really a healing power that exists within you? Absolutely! The first place you need to look is at the source of this power, which is in your body's own field of energy. Let me explain how it works.

There are many forms of energy surrounding us every day. We turn on our televisions, boot up our computers, recharge our smart phones, and turn on our car headlights without thinking twice about the electrical energy that powers it all. There is also the type of energy you probably feel surge through you when you eat your quinoa and kale, or even when you devour your pizza and ice cream. Then there's the solar energy that warms this great planet of ours, and the wind energies that we hope will someday replace the power now provided by fossil fuels and nuclear power plants.

The energy that is the source of your healing power is similar to these forms of energy. This energy is a living force within you that originates both inside

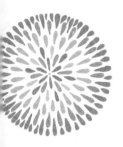

and outside of you. You may already know several names for it. The Hindus call it *prana*, the Chinese call it *chi*, and the Japanese call it *qi*. It's within you right now—invisible streams of get-up-and-go flowing through all of your body's energy channels or meridians.

This primal force of energy is connected to your spirit as well as to your physical, emotional, and mental bodies. In fact, it's the *substance* of spirit. I like to call this LifeForce Energy because it combines the powerful energies of your personal energy field and the universal energy field, which includes everyone and everything.

Once you understand how you and the rest of the world run on this universal field of energy, you'll be able to learn how to use your innate power to tap into this field. You'll be able to harness this energy and use it to activate any changes you desire. Perhaps you want to heal a part of your body, fix a relationship, or deepen your spirituality. You can plug into this energy to get answers to your deepest questions. You may even want to train further in how to manage this energy by becoming an energy healer who helps humanity at large.

Now, before you make the decision to develop this vibrant gift that lies within you, I'd like to share a little about my personal story and how I first learned about this very powerful gift that transformed my life.

How I Discovered My Innate Power to Heal

I discovered my own innate power to heal when I was smacked hard by a traumatic event in my mid-twenties. One day everything seemed to be going well, and the next day my doctor brought my life to a standstill. She said the words no one wants to hear: "You have cancer."

I had cervical cancer.

Looking back, it seems that the trouble started in my tumultuous childhood, growing up in a home with a family member who sexually abused me. I didn't know how to handle all of the emotions I was feeling, so I began to bury them under a thick shadow of addictions and behaviors of acting out. From the time I

was a teenager to a young adult, I used alcohol, drugs, and a risk-taking lifestyle to deal with my pain.

When I was in my early twenties, I was a workaholic, fresh out of law school and trying cases. I was an athlete, drawn to extreme sports like mountain climbing and ski racing, and at times I was a model, which meant maintaining a size 2 body. My life was go, go, go—fueled by cigarettes and booze, Valium and diet soda. I always kept my attention directed anywhere other than my inner pain. I didn't want to talk about it. I didn't want to think about it. And I certainly didn't want anybody to know about it. I just wanted it to go away.

Then came that shocking diagnosis: cancer.

At the time, medical options for cervical cancer were grim, with all fingers pointing to radical surgery. I knew in my gut there had to be another way to beat it, so I went to my doctors and asked how much time I had before I had to make a decision. They gave me the window of a few months. That was all I needed to hear.

Right away I knew I had to clean up my act—namely my addictions. The first item on my agenda was to find a 12-step program. I lived in a tiny town where everyone knew everyone else's business. Of course, the last thing I wanted was for anyone in the community to know that I had a drinking problem. No one around me, not even my closest business partners, knew (or so I kidded myself). I still remember getting ready to go to that first meeting. Like most alcoholics, I wanted to look like I had it together, so I got dressed to the teeth for the gathering, even donning a flashy pair of cowboy boots. I walked into the room and couldn't believe what I saw. Right away, I recognized three other local lawyers. "Oh, I didn't know..." They looked quite amused. "Well, we didn't know about you either." At the first meeting I attended, I rediscovered my spiritual roots when they said the Serenity Prayer. As a Catholic child, I had a deep connection to Jesus and the saints, so it wasn't hard to reestablish my connection to the Divine, which I had shut down as a teenager.

Once alcohol and Valium were out of the picture, I wanted to get in touch with my emotions, sensing that they were connected to the cancer. I had buried them for so long, they were screaming inside me to be released. I knew that in order to heal, I had to find them. I started to take note of what I was feeling, even jotting

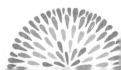

down words in the margins of my legal briefs to put a name to my emotions as I experienced them. *Jealousy. Anger. Fear. Shame.* I had a lot more going on inside than I had realized.

Figuring I had to look within more closely, I began to meditate—a practice I have expanded and built upon and continue to this day. I also took up journaling, and that's when the pain of my childhood poured out (parts of my journal from that time wound up in my first bestselling book, *Truth Heals*).

As part of my healing journey, I began seeing practitioners for acupuncture and massage. It was then that I first heard about energy medicine. I had visited a new massage therapist, and at the end of the session, out of the blue she said, "You could benefit from energy healing. I'm going to give you a referral. Call her." I couldn't sleep when I went to bed that night. A strong vibration kept me awake for the next few nights.

I called the referral number and then drove three hours to see the energy healer. When the healer walked into the waiting room, she was dressed like I was, in a business suit and pearls. Highly intuitive, she had purposely dressed like that to put me at ease. I had an amazing transformation during the next hour on her table. I could feel her focused energy. It calmed and renewed my spirit. For the first time in longer than I could remember, I felt a sense of peace as though she had healed my emotional turmoil and my spirit. This in turn gave my body the strength and support it needed to fight the cancer. At the third session with the energy healer, I felt a major shift in my body and sensed healing. The very next day, I returned to my medical doctor for tests and was informed that no further medical intervention was necessary—I had undergone a "spontaneous remission." I knew that I owed my remission to the power of energy healing.

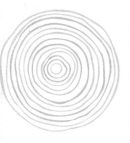

At that point I wanted to know more about this amazing power, so I began what would turn into decades of study and training with shamans, sages, and healers from every walk of life, from esoteric Christians in the West, to seers in the East, to shamanic traditions from Native American and South American cultures. I wanted to know anything and everything about this healing force. I wanted to use this healing energy in my own life as well as share it with others so they too could heal.

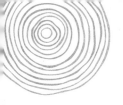

Over the years I became a teacher of energy healing and developed a technique of my own. I've shared this knowledge in my workshops, lectures, and online classes. But I wanted to do more. I knew in my heart that this gift of energy healing was something that everyone could embrace. I wanted to shout this message out to the world!

That's why I'm writing this book—to give you the ultimate guide on how you can activate your internal healing power and use it to enrich your own life as well as the lives of the people around you. Just like the proverbial stone thrown into the pond that creates ever-expanding circles in the water, the power of energy healing can be multiplied in healing circles to expand out and heal the world.

What's Your Story?

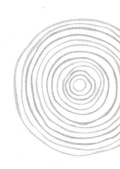

Perhaps you have buried a traumatic event of your life and you're having trouble keeping those unpleasant emotions bottled inside. Maybe you've been experiencing anxiety or insomnia or inexplicable weight gain. Or maybe your doctor says you have diabetes or high blood pressure or asthma and wants to put you on a course of medical treatment complete with side effects and no recovery in sight.

Maybe you're just sick and tired of being sick and tired. The world is sucking you dry. You're at your wit's end about how to go about changing your life. You're not sure if finding another partner, another job, another doctor, or another place to live is the answer. You're anxious, depressed, angry, or perhaps bingeing on anything that will give you some temporary relief. You can stop the self-destructive behaviors, the self-pity, the feeling that you're stuck. You are capable of breaking free and bursting forward into a better life.

Today's medical system has splintered into specialty after specialty. Experts may be very proficient at addressing specific symptoms, usually with a major assist from the pharmaceutical industry, but they don't always look at the entire picture or address you as a whole person. They don't tend to explore the emotional, psychological, and spiritual components that can contribute to or even cause your problems. That's where energy medicine comes in.

Energy Healing Will Change Your Life

Energy healing can improve your life on every level—physical, psychological, emotional, and spiritual. I know that may sound like a pretty bold statement, but it's true. When you start to clear away the emotional debris you've stored in your energy field and learn how to bring higher vibratory energies into yourself, a brighter, healthier, and happier life can be yours.

You will have more awareness of your own being—from your physical body to your connection to the entire universe—and be able to make the changes you need, without fearing change itself. Energy healing will work on your whole being, using natural, nontoxic techniques to help heal or prevent physical symptoms from developing. And when you activate your inner power, you can learn to do a lot of this energy healing on yourself. Your health, your finances, your relationships, your emotional stability, and even your environment can improve!

That being said, I also believe that it's important to work with the medical world and other experts in their respective fields. If you're sick—that is, if the problem has manifested as disease in your physical body—you definitely want Western medical help along with complementary or alternative approaches. I encourage you to get everyone on board: embrace the knowledge, wisdom, and skills of your entire medical team.

When you activate the healing energy that is lying dormant inside of you, you will discover that you have many more options for healing and changing your life. That's what energy healing does: it takes into account your whole being and sees the interconnections between your body and mind, heart and soul.

EMBRACE AND EXPAND
YOUR ENERGY

magine that you have just arrived at your favorite seaside retreat for a short weekend break. You immediately walk out to the beach, kicking off your shoes as you step onto the warm sand, stopping where the water reaches the shore. As you look out over the ocean, the sea breeze gently blows a few strands of hair across your face. You hear wave after wave crash onto the shore and watch as each wave buries your bare feet deeper in the cool, wet sand. You inhale the briny odor of the ocean and taste the salty drops of seawater that have splashed on your face. The air is warm and humid, caressing your skin. In the distance, the white sail of a boat stands out against the cerulean blue of the sky. You remember when you used to come here as a child and can feel again the sense of wonder and joy that enveloped you here. *Ahhh.* Heaven.

This hypothetical reveals how you can use all of your senses to feel the energy that is around you and within you. Your five basic senses—sight, sound, smell, taste, and touch—are the gateways to explore your physical reality. The universal energy field comes to us through our environment and from the people we are in touch with. Sometimes the field feels as serene as the beach on a crystal-clear day. Other times it can be harsh or jarring. If you're at that beautiful beach on a perfectly awesome day and suddenly someone yells, "Shark!" the energetic charge of fear can ruin your good mood and set your feet in motion to hightail it out of there.

Beyond what you can experience through your physical senses, there is a sixth sense—intuition: the "gut feeling" that colors your perceptions. Maybe while standing at that beach and having your toes tickled by the ocean water as it hits the shore, you suddenly have an uneasy feeling, like something isn't quite right, even in this paradise. Then someone shouts, "Shark!" Even though you were not consciously aware of the shark's presence, you could somehow sense the danger. That's your intuitive sense knowing something is off-kilter.

Get to Know Your Personal Energy Field

Your personal energy field consists of the energy that flows through and around your body. This energy field can also be called your aura, as it gives out electromagnetic energy and radiates light.

Your personal energy field has seven main energy centers. You might know these as your chakras. The word *chakra* stems from Sanskrit and means "wheel" or "circle." These source points of spinning energy are composed of bundles of nerves; they connect to some of your major organs and glands, and they house your emotional and spiritual energies.

The seven main chakras are like a totem pole, going from the base of your spine to the top of your head: the first, or base chakra, is connected to survival and the health of your body; the second, or sacral chakra, is home to the pleasure principle and the seat of your creativity; the third, or solar plexus chakra, is the furnace of your power and will; the fourth is the heart chakra and the seat of love for the self; the fifth chakra, at the throat, is the center of expression; the "third eye," or sixth, chakra holds the energy of spiritual insight and intuition; and the seventh, or crown, chakra is the radiant center of higher "knowing" and connection to Source.

Your chakras can reveal a lot about you. The lower three chakras tip you off about the safety and survival of your physical body, your relationship with yourself and others, and your personal power. The fourth chakra, the heart, is the point of balance in the whole system; it connects the lower three chakras with the upper three chakras that are the spiritual centers that connect you to Source. If there is any imbalance or distortion in your energy field, your chakras will certainly let you know, and eventually your physical body will reflect what is happening in your energy field.

How you navigate the world is directly dependent on the way your chakras or energy centers are working. For example, Marilyn Monroe's energy was predominantly in the second chakra; the main way in which she saw the world and acted in it was through her sensuality. Napoleon Bonaparte operated predominately out of the third chakra—power and will—while Martin Luther King Jr. approached life principally from his throat chakra. Someone like the Dalai Lama has powerful energy in the seventh chakra.

Chakra Check Using a Penduluma

In order to activate your energy healing ability, you need to *experience* the human energy field. One of the best ways to do this is by using a pendulum. This is a simple device that responds to the otherwise imperceptible movement of nearby energy. Anyone can

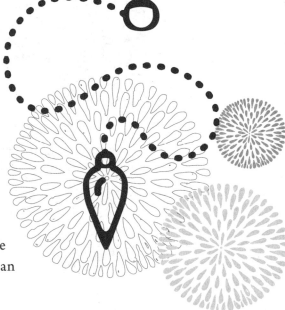

use this powerful tool; it just takes practice, like learning a musical instrument. A pendulum is a simple object suspended on a chain or cord, which can help you locate a chakra or energy center as well as determine its movement. When you hold a pendulum directly over a chakra, it will move in the direction of the energy flow coming from that chakra.

Pendulums can be made out of a wide variety of materials, including crystal, glass, various metals, and wood. In my experience, the most effective and safe pendulums for testing your chakras are made out of beechwood and are conical in shape. Crystal and metal pendulums are popular items in many bookstores and specialty shops these days, but they take a lot of training to use and can "cut" a chakra, damaging it energetically, so save them for much later.

When you first get your pendulum, I recommend carrying it around with you in a pocket, purse, or backpack for a few days so it begins to resonate with your energy. One of the most powerful ways to clear and recharge your pendulum is to place it outside during dry weather when there's a full moon. Finally, it's best not to loan your pendulum to others, unless it's so they can test *your* chakras.

Exercise: Checking Your Personal Energy Field

Here's an exercise to check your energy centers. You'll need a pendulum, a close friend, and the illustration of chakra locations (see page 10). Have your friend lie down on her back, preferably on a hard surface like a kitchen counter or massage table rather than on a couch or bed. Stand above her as you hold the pendulum four to six inches above one of the chakras, being careful not to let the pendulum touch her body. After a moment, the pendulum will begin to move. Give it about ten seconds for the movement to settle firmly into a pattern. The hard part is keeping your mind free of any expectations about what the pendulum will reveal.

After you test your friend's chakras, have her test yours. Keep an open mind about the results, since you are both new at this. Note that the way the pendulum is spinning is from the perspective of the person who is holding the pendulum. Here's what the movement means when it's over a chakra:

- *Clockwise* movement indicates open, well-balanced energy.

- *Counterclockwise* movement indicates a possible blockage in that chakra or negativity that needs to be cleared.

- *No movement* at all indicates a closed chakra.

- An *elliptical* swing indicates an imbalance in the way the energy is flowing. The more distorted the movement is, the more severe the distortion of that chakra.

- The *size of the circle* that the pendulum makes can indicate how much energy is flowing through the chakra; ideally, the size is similar among all your chakras.

To give you a better idea as to how this exercise works, I'd like to share an experience I had with a chakra reading. Back in the days when I was still seeing private clients, Maria came to me with pain in her upper back. While sensing her chakras and then checking them with a pendulum, I could see that her lower chakras were all normal, while her fourth chakra was "dead in the water," meaning it was 100 percent closed. She'd had a relationship go sour and, like so many people when they get hurt, had shut down her heart chakra. The chakras project your feelings and beliefs to the world. If a chakra is moving in the wrong direction or is closed, it signals a distortion in your energy and means that the message you send out to the world can be equally distorted. In the case of a closed heart chakra, the message sent is often "I'm not worthy of love." This practically guarantees that you are not going to be open to a new relationship, no matter how much you say you want one.

I helped Maria balance and recalibrate her heart chakra, and I guided her to let go of her feelings of resentment toward her ex. Her heart chakra righted itself. Some weeks later, Maria came back, and her back pain was a thing of the past. I could sense that Maria would soon meet someone and be open to a new relationship.

At one time or another, each and every one of us will experience blockages in our energy field and chakras. It is up to you to become aware of your own energy field, how energy is flowing through it, and when and where it is blocked. In the process of reading this book, you will begin to gain that awareness. The most powerful way to bolster and sustain your health is by constantly bringing universal energy through your chakras, into your field, and into your body. This dynamic exchange between the universal field and your personal energy field will make you a powerhouse of good health!

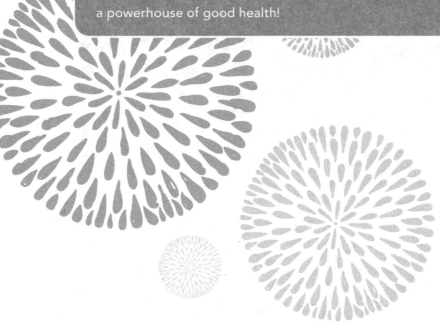

POWER UP YOUR BODY

Good health is all about internal balance and dynamic interplay with the environment. That means your energy is in balance and flowing smoothly and that you're exchanging energy and interacting with all the people and situations surrounding you in a harmonious way. It's when your energy becomes stuck, static, or blocked that you get emotionally off-balance or even sick.

Suppose you lose a parent and instead of giving yourself a chance to grieve adequately, you simply repress those feelings, go to the funeral, and head back to work on Monday. You push your real feelings down somewhere in your body and psyche, where they start festering. A month, a year, five years, or decades later, you may find yourself dealing with a full-blown disease process that originated from the blockage of that grief. Our postmodern culture does not teach us how to deal with negative emotions, and their lower vibrations stay lodged in our energy field and body where, sooner or later, they can wreak havoc if they remain unprocessed.

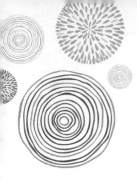

Everything Vibrates

You are a vibratory being—you are constantly sending out your unique vibration. Your energy field is constantly receiving outside vibrations, and interacting with everyone and everything around you. You take in and respond to the pulsations of energy in your environment. When you were a teen, your mother might have said something like "If you hang around with those losers, you're going to wind up like them!" She was sensing your energy field when you came home after being around those kids; your energy field had lowered itself to match their vibration.

Everything vibrates. The components of your physical body—your cells, your organs, your internal systems (digestion, breathing, and so on)—all vibrate at their own rate. Your consciousness has its own vibration. The faster the vibration, the higher the consciousness. A wall vibrates so slowly that you think of it as solid. Yet I have learned of masters from the East, now long gone, who could raise their vibration to such a high pitch that they could indeed walk through walls.[1] For a recent example, consider Padre Pio, a humble Italian priest who died in the 1960s. He was known for levitating, permanent visible stigmata, and according to eyewitnesses he could bilocate, or be in two places at the same time.[2]

A key point to keep in mind is that your body grows out of your energy field, not the other way around. Before your physical body manifests and you take birth on earth, your body first becomes organized in the higher energetic dimensions as an etheric template—the design for who you will be and the lessons you are here to learn. Now that you are here in a body, if something's showing up in your field that isn't optimal, like a blockage or a distortion, you can work on it on the energetic levels *before* it manifests on the physical plane and shows up as a disease in your body.

The Levels of the Field

The human energy field is much more complex than you can imagine. It is composed of seven main levels that interpenetrate one another and your body. Each level of the field is a higher vibration and extends out from your body farther than those below it. This is what forms your aura—the luminous radiation that surrounds you and can be sensed with a little training.

Levels one, three, five, and seven—the odd-numbered levels—look like lines of light. Levels two, four, and six are more formless, composed of cloudlike energy that can have different colors and densities. The "clouds" of the even-numbered levels seem to be held together by the more structured odd-numbered levels. Together, all the levels of the human energy field communicate with one another to supply you and your body with life energy.

If any of these levels are insufficiently charged, or aren't strong enough, your experiences in life may be disappointing. You might wind up with a physical problem if a level is out of sync for an extended period of time. Your body arises from your energy field, which means that imbalances or distortions in the field will eventually impact your body in a negative way. Of course, if you correct those imbalances, your body will respond in a positive way. When you adjust the energy field, you can often prevent a potential illness from showing up in your body. That is why frequently restructuring, rebalancing, and charging the field are so important.

Here are the levels:

The etheric level: This is the level that's closest to your body, only a few inches out from your skin. As an uneven number, this level is composed of structured lines of bright-blue light. Here is where you feel the physical sensations of pain and pleasure. If you are active physically, the first level will be strong. If you are not as physically active, the lines will look thinner, finer, and be a lighter shade of blue. The better care you take of your body, the stronger this level will be and the more you will enjoy feelings of physical pleasure. Your body likes to have physical contact with its inner and outer environment through activities like eating, smelling, tasting, watching, walking, dancing, and swimming. Issues can arise if your first level is weak—for instance, if you like to eat but hate to move your body in physical exercise.

How would you rate the strength of your first level? Do you move your body for at least an hour a day, or do you spend all day sitting in front of

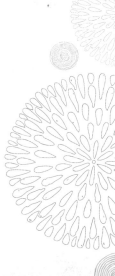

a computer followed by an evening sitting in front of the television? Do you enjoy physical touch, or do you shy away from being hugged? Think of ways you could connect more strongly with your physical body.

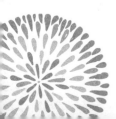 **The emotional level:** This cloudlike level shows how you feel about yourself. The brighter the colors on this level, the more positive you feel about yourself; darker colors indicate a negative self-image. If you allow your emotions to flow through you, rather than repressing or blocking them, the colors are in motion and keep changing. However, if you hold on to an emotion, like anger or fear, the flow stops and this level gets stagnant, which creates blockages that can damage your health not just on this level but also on the adjacent first and third levels. If this level is dark or stagnant, you don't like yourself very much—an unhealthy state of affairs that needs to be addressed.

To evaluate yourself on this level, ask: Am I in touch with my feelings? How do I feel about myself? Has self-esteem or self-acceptance always been an issue for me? Am I okay with the way I process my emotions?

The mental level: Extending another inch or two out past the second level, this one is about your mind. Strong lines here indicate an active and clear mind, while weak and undercharged lines mean you probably don't have a lot of clarity and might not be that interested in learning. If your first two levels are weak but this one is strong, you may live mostly in your head. In today's culture, where you are more likely to be sitting at a desk doing mental work than to be out farming the land, that's a very common situation.

Do you believe that the way to solve your problems is by using your reasoning capacity rather than by being in touch with your physical and emotional needs? Are most of your activities mental (reading, watching television, playing video games, being online) or do you also enjoy gardening, working out, dancing, playing music, or painting?

The astral level: This level is all about your relationship with others—all the people, animals, flora and fauna, and even the inanimate objects of Earth, as well as the planets, solar system, and the whole universe. This level feels like thick liquid, and if it is undercharged with a low vibration, the fluid may feel thick and dark, and you might experience pain, exhaustion, and eventually disease. Some writers refer to the fourth level energy as "bioplasma," which sends out streamers of beautiful colors between two people who love or feel good about each other. Love streamers are pink or light-red waves, while dark-red streamers indicate anger and green ones indicate envy.

If this level is strong and healthy, you'll have great relationships. To evaluate this level, ask yourself: Do I avoid intimacy? Do I choose to spend a lot of my time alone? Am I not all that interested in other people? If so, your fourth level may be weak. If that's the case, remember that everything is about self-awareness. Be gentle with yourself.

The etheric template: Now we're on the level of divine will, which looks just like a blueprint of the first level—the form for your body. It extends about a foot or two out from your body. This is the level of the spiritual guides (see chapter 11) and of pure intention, which is why it's the perfect level for energy healing. Here you find precise order and symbols, not feelings. If you're in sync with divine will, you'll feel connected with the world around you, and you'll sense that you're on the right path in the right place at the right time. If this level is weak, you may feel disconnected, like you don't fit in, and you are probably not comfortable with your place, your job, or your life in general.

Do you feel like you're on the right path? Do you feel a sense of belonging? Do the events in your life reflect your connection to divine will?

The celestial body: This is the level of divine love, which extends two or three feet out from your body and has within it every color of

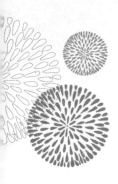

the rainbow in beautiful streamers of light. It's a high frequency, so when this level is healthy and well developed, the colors are bright with straight beams of light and you can have blissful spiritual experiences. If the sixth level is too weak or undercharged, you may be lacking spiritual training or might have experienced some sort of spiritual trauma. If it's too strong compared to other levels of the field, you may be distorting this level to avoid life on the physical plane. That is not a good scenario, since you need the vehicle of the body for this lifetime. This level gets depleted every day and needs to be recharged, which can be done with simply twenty minutes of meditation a day.

Are you having spiritual experiences? Do you sometimes feel joy when you meditate or pray or chant? Remember to recharge this level with your meditation practice.

The ketheric template (or causal body): This level is composed of gold lines that vibrate at a very high frequency to form a golden egg of protection all around you. It extends around three to four feet from your body and holds your whole field together. This is the level of divine mind, where you access truth, are able to communicate telepathically, and have "knowings" about others or yourself that flood your consciousness. A healthy seventh level gives you a strong sense of your place in the world, and you will be able to carry out important concepts for how to move the world in a positive direction. You're a "big" thinker, connected with divine thought. If this level is not healthy, it will be filled with lines that are dull or visually weak, or may even be torn. That usually indicates a perfectionist who is unwilling to accept any human imperfections in themselves.

Do you have trouble manifesting your creative ideas? Are you super hard on yourself? Do you accept your own human failings? Think about it.

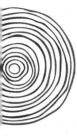

Now that you have the big picture of the human energy field, it's time to learn more about the chakras, the energy centers that are the focal points in your human energy field.

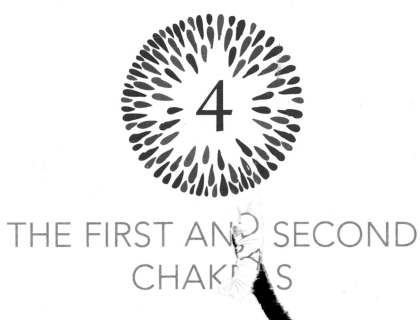

THE FIRST AND SECOND CHAKRAS

Your inner healing power runs on energy. That energy is concentrated in seven main power centers that are in your personal energy field and are called chakras.

Your chakras start at the base of your spine and go right to the top of your head. The seven main chakras are: (1) the root, or base chakra, connected to survival and safety; (2) the sacral chakra, home to the pleasure principle of attraction and desire; (3) the solar plexus chakra, the furnace of your personal power and the seat of your self-esteem; (4) the heart chakra, the seat of self-love and compassion for others; it bridges the lower three chakras and the upper three; (5) the throat chakra, the center of communication and expression; (6) the "third eye," with the energy of insight and intuition; and (7) the crown chakra, your radiant spiritual center and connection to Source.

Your personal energy field flows through and congregates around these seven energy centers. When your chakras are open, your energy flows easily and freely. But if someone messes with you emotionally and psychologically—maybe a parent who embarrasses you in front of your friends or a partner who has lost interest in you—and if you hold on to that experience rather than process it, it can cause a blockage that prevents your energy from flowing.

During the next several chapters, I'm going to teach you all about your chakras, how they speak up when there's trouble, how to clear up any blockages that can eventually turn into physical ailments, and what you can do to keep your energy healthy and flowing strong. I'll also give you information on the archetypes connected to each chakra, their spiritual significance, and their astrological associations.

Each chakra plays a central role in your health and well-being. Let's begin with the first two energy centers—survival and movement.

The First Chakra—Survival

Before you can put your energy to work for yourself, others, or the world, you have to explore the roots of your past and learn the reason for your existence.

The instinct for survival is the key to the first chakra, located at the base of the spine. It is also called the base chakra or the root chakra because it's your connection to the earth as well as the support beam for all the chakras above it. Every chakra has a governing principle: for this chakra, it's *foundation*. In Sanskrit,

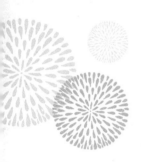

the first chakra is called the *muladhara*, which means "root support."

A healthy first chakra is red, vibrant, humming, and open. It has volcanic energy from Mother Earth, coming from the earth up through the soles of your feet, up your legs, and right into this first chakra. It makes you want to stay here on earth. It's your connection to your physical body and your health. When energy flows freely in the first chakra, it keeps you feeling safe, secure, grounded, and present.

The first chakra relates to the element of earth and builds the structure that supports and sustains your life. Think of how your legs and feet root you to the earth. The sciatic nerve, which even looks like a root system, starts near the first chakra and goes down to your feet, connecting your nervous system to the ground beneath you. It's the constant tug of gravity that keeps you grounded. Roots have both masculine and feminine powers: they penetrate the earth, pushing down into the soil, and they are receptive, bringing up nourishment from the earth. When you're able to "hold your ground" and be receptive to getting support and nourishment, you have a solid foundation.

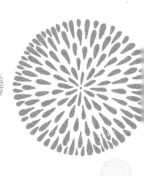

The First Chakra's Biggest Obstacle

When you don't feel secure, when you don't feel like you "belong" here on earth, when you are disconnected from your physical body and the natural world, you lose energy and start to worry about your existence. Fear, which is the biggest obstacle to free-flowing energy in the first chakra, can come in many forms: fear about your personal safety, about not fitting in with your family or friends or where you live, about your job and money issues, about being alone, even about death.

The Health of Your First Chakra

You know you have a balanced first chakra if you are centered and grounded, you take care of your body, and you have a sense of being fully alive. When your energy is flowing easily through your first chakra, you have a powerful will to live a healthy life. The earth element nourishes your bones, blood, muscles, and even the hair on your body. Earth is the densest of all the elements and provides stability and security for your existence through your base chakra. The nose is the sense organ for this chakra, since the sense of smell is related to the element of earth. Now you know why you feel so great when you walk under a fragrant pine tree.

Problems with the first chakra can originate in the womb, with the fetus absorbing the fear and anxiety of the mother, or during the birth process itself, especially if it was a difficult one. Lack of bonding with your mother for any reason can also create a very shaky foundation.

The key issues for this chakra are concerned with the safety and survival of your body: trust, nourishment, health, home, family, and tribe. When something is going wrong in one of these areas of your life, it can affect your first chakra. Situations that can wreak havoc on your first chakra include any kind of abuse, surgeries, major illnesses or accidents, natural disasters, violence, job loss, a change in housing, or abandonment by a parent, partner, or caregiver.

Problems in this chakra typically show up at the base of your spine, in your legs and feet, in your bones, or in your immune system. They may also manifest as eating disorders, adrenal insufficiency, or rectal or colon cancer.

The governing glands of the first chakra are the adrenals, even though they aren't located anywhere near the base chakra. The first chakra is all about survival; when your food, shelter, safety, or sleep is threatened, your adrenal glands kick in to give you the burst of energy you need to escape the situation.

Archetypes

In the Western psychological tradition, chakras can be looked at through the lens of archetypes. Carl G. Jung, the noted Swiss psychiatrist, created the psychological concept of Jungian archetypes, which develop from the collective unconscious; they can be recognized by the patterns of behavior that are projected out of our strengths and weaknesses, our positive and negative qualities.

The dysfunctional archetype for the first chakra is the victim, and the functional archetype is that of the Earth Mother. The victim is a low level of consciousness and energy. Victims are sure that someone or something external causes everything that happens in their lives; therefore, their fate is not in their control. You can become a victim when you lose your grounding and everything seems to be a constant struggle. You can't connect with your inner core, so your spirit can't fly high. With no sense of personal empowerment, you get stuck in fear of what will come at you from outside. When you once again get grounded, get connected back to your body and the earth, you can accept that you may indeed be responsible for what is happening in your life and that you might have to make some changes within yourself.

The positive archetype, the Earth Mother, represents your ability to be in charge of your own life force. The Earth Mother, rooted as she is in the energy of the earth, is a reliable source of nourishment that can provide you with whatever you need. When you can mother yourself, your life will be in balance.

Spiritual Aspects

The chakra system originated many thousands of years ago from Vedic philosophy, and the ancient seers who codified the system recognized the connection of the chakras to Spirit. Each chakra is connected to Source, and each of the seven main chakras in the body has a seed syllable sound, a presiding deity, and a connection to a particular planet.

The root chakra is the resting place of *kundalini*, the energy of consciousness, which is represented as a snake that is coiled and sleeping at the base of the spine. Before this energy can awaken, you have to open and clear the first chakra. All the other chakras can receive only as much energy as the flow generated in the first chakra. This is why all physical illness has a strong relationship to the first chakra.

For the first chakra, the seed sound is *Lam*. Repetition of this sound as a mantra gives you a greater connection to the element of earth and great inner strength. Airavata is an elephant, the symbol of strength that carries the seed sound. An elephant can carry heavy loads yet is also humble in carrying out its master's orders, indicating that spiritual strength can be in harmony with good strong physical health.

Brahma, the Hindu deity who is the creator of the physical plane, is the ruler of the root chakra. The symbol for the first chakra is a four-petal lotus, just as Brahma is depicted as having four heads representing the four aspects of human consciousness—the physical, emotional, rational, and intuitive. Before you invoke

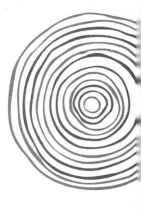

Lord Brahma to help you open and clear your first chakra (or before invoking any other deity), you should invoke Ganesh first, as he removes any obstacles and bestows protection at the beginning of any undertaking. This elephant-headed deity was created by Parvati from the clay of her own body, which is how Ganesh is connected to the element of earth, the element of the first chakra. Parvati is also the wife of Lord Shiva, who is one of the principal deities in the Hindu faith, a supreme being that creates the universe.

I'd like to add a note here about the deities. Westerners are often confused by the great array of gods and goddesses in the Hindu and Tibetan Buddhist traditions, and they may worry that invoking one or more of these deities is somehow antithetical to their own religious beliefs. Be assured that even though these many gods all have distinct looks and personalities, they are all aspects of *Brahman*, the one ultimate reality, which is within every living being. They represent different aspects of consciousness and, as such, are very helpful when you want to focus your attention in a particular direction.

Astrologically, the planets of Saturn and Earth are connected to the base chakra. Saturn has a bad rap for causing delays and for the hard work needed to surmount the challenges it brings, but it is also a strict but wise teacher that will advance you along the spiritual path. You might want to check your birth chart to see where Saturn sits in your chart. If it's in a difficult placement, it may block your first chakra energy. However, any type of consistent physical exercise, like hatha yoga, will offset Saturn's placement.

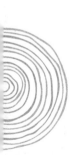

Know When to Give Your First Chakra a Tune-Up

When I was young, I was restless and anxious, the result of post-traumatic stress from my abusive childhood. As a teenager and later when I was in my twenties, I had an eating disorder and nagging lower leg and knee pain. My first (and second) chakras were basically shut down, which explains why I ended up with cervical cancer at such a young age. I helped address this issue with energy healing that cleared the effects of the original trauma and also with healthy practices like Pilates to get me back in touch with my body.

Even if you are not currently experiencing negative health effects, it is a good idea to periodically check your first chakra to make sure it is healthy. To do this, answer these questions honestly:

- Do you have a hard time staying focused?
- Are you excessively fearful?
- Do you have any phobias?
- Are you taking medication for anxiety?
- Are your desk, your household, or your finances disorganized?
- Do you feel too weak for sustained physical activity?
- Are you very uncomfortable when things change?
- Are you often doing one thing while thinking about another?

If you answered yes to three or more of these questions, chances are your first chakra could use a tune-up.

How to Clear First Chakra Blockages

There are multiple ways that you can help heal your first chakra. For example, since the color of the first chakra is red—symbolizing the blood of life, vitality, and our physical nature—most red stones relate to the root chakra. Garnet, bloodstone, ruby, red jasper, coral, and rose quartz can all provide a healing vibration for the first chakra. You can hold a stone in the palm of your hand while you bring its energy into your field, or you can put the stone on a table near your meditation seat and visualize the red energy entering and healing your first chakra. If you have an altar, you can also place the stone there.

When trying to heal your first chakra, you should try to eat lots of protein because it's good for grounding. When you feel weak or out of touch with your body and the physical world, root vegetables and flesh food, including small portions of organic grass-fed beef, can act as a foundation to keep the first chakra healthy. Be careful, though—too much protein can make you feel sluggish, and that doesn't work when you're trying to help yourself, others, or the world.

Healing can take place in the first chakra when you reestablish a connection to physical reality, whether through spending time outside in nature with Mother Earth or through any practice that puts you more in touch with your body. You might try martial arts, yoga, or Pilates to help you get more grounded. To balance your first chakra, you could also use cedar incense or essential oil of cedar; its woodsy smell will remind you of a tree supported by a strong network of roots.

Other simple ways to clear your first chakra are walking barefoot, hiking in the park or in the mountains, dancing, belly breathing, gardening, creating order and structure in your house, wearing the color red, and repeating affirmations like *I have a right to be here and I am safe.*

First Chakra Exercise: The Practice of Presence

Perhaps you're worrying about paying the bills, whether your kids will get into the right schools, or if you'll ever meet the soul mate of your dreams. That's living in the future. Perhaps you're fretting over injustices you suffered in a less than amicable divorce or an argument you had with your mother just before she died. That's living in the past.

It's better to *live in the present*, where you will find yourself much calmer and happier, taking one moment at a time. Living in the moment is the best way to sustain your first chakra. Pay attention to cutting those vegetables rather than worrying about your to-do list as you chop that carrot. Walk outside without your smart phone and just absorb the sounds, smells, and sights of the natural world. Take a moment to stretch and feel your body, breathing into areas of stiffness or pain.

Can you live in the present moment? Try doing something that will bolster and support your first chakra today. See how much better you feel being present in the here and now.

The Second Chakra—Movement

The second chakra is the center of your pleasure principle; it's about you in relation to others, about attraction and desire. The governing principle of the second chakra is about the movement of the body and its connection to others. This center is sometimes called the sacral chakra because it's located halfway between the base chakra and the navel, corresponding to the sacral plexus nerve ganglion that connects to the sciatic nerve. The second chakra is a vivid orange, and it's all about your emotions and your childhood. It's your creative center, whether it's art, music, writing, your work or hobbies, sports—anything. In Sanskrit, it is called the *swadhisthana*, which means "sweetness." What could be sweeter than being creative and feeling pleasure? When the roots of the first chakra are strong, they can support a plant that gives sweet fruit. When you reach the higher levels of meditation, a sweet honeylike taste comes into your mouth and a warm, tingling rush comes up your spine.

The second chakra relates to the element of water. Here you move from standing on the solid ground of your first chakra to the fluid world of your second chakra. This chakra is the essence of life as seen in bodily fluids like blood and tears and lymph. There is no life on earth without water. While the first chakra challenges you to create structure and hold your ground, the second wants you to let go so your creativity can flow. As the foundation of your emotional body and the center of the pleasure principle, it allows you to *feel* your emotions, to be open and friendly with other people, and to be in touch with your sexuality and sensuality.

I'd like to add a note here about sexuality. The West has always been on shaky ground about sexuality, seeing it frequently as forbidden and wrong. The East sees it differently.

The chakra system was derived from Tantric philosophy, which honors the body as being sacred. This is based on seeing the universe as having manifested from the divine Source that creates and preserves the universe, and thus everything in it must be sacred. Tantra teaches that you can reach enlightenment through your body's senses. Tantric practices range far beyond sex, including the recognition that you and the deity you are worshipping are the same in essence. Tantra uses *mantras* (sacred sounds), *mudras* (hand gestures), *yantras* (mystical diagrams), and *mandalas* (geometric patterns that represent the universe) to enlighten through the senses. As His Holiness the Dalai Lama said, "In brief, the body of a Buddha is attained through meditating on it."[1]

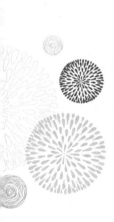

So what is tantric sex? Throughout East Indian art and mythology are images of sexual union, with the male representing pure consciousness that becomes activated when it joins together with the feminine *shakti*, divine energy. Tantric sexual practices use the controlled energy of sexual arousal to awaken the sleeping kundalini and raise that energy up the spine. True adepts of these practices can elevate their consciousness through refined sexual control practices to achieve the highest level of *samadhi*. However, don't go rushing out to buy a book or go online to learn tantric sexual practices; they are really for those who are advanced in consciousness and no longer attached to the personal dramas of relationships.

The Second Chakra's Biggest Obstacle

When your chakras are distorted, they can have either too much or too little energy. When there is too much energy in the second chakra, you may be too emotional and find yourself caught in anger or jealousy or rage. This chakra is also where one of the biggest problems shows up—addiction. Addictions range from alcohol, drugs, food, shopping, exercise, sex, gambling, and pornography to spending way too much time on video games or social media.

The Health of Your Second Chakra

A healthy second chakra enables you to find the balance between giving and receiving. You're able to appreciate the material things in your life, such as your home, car, clothes, and electronics, but you shop wisely. You know how to balance your work life and social life, and you often feel happy and excited about new creative projects—such as concocting a delicious new recipe or redecorating a room in your home. You don't try to control others, and you can grasp the consequences of your actions. You can identify any unhealthy addictive patterns you may have and find a way to change them.

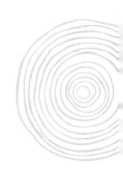

The main themes of the second chakra are trust and faith, which rely more on feelings than on linear thinking. As a result, life situations involving negative emotions are most likely to cause problems with your second chakra. Some of these include feeling guilt about having sex or receiving pleasure, burying your anger, engaging in addictive behavior, experiencing your parents' divorce when you were a child, losing a parent at a young age, or being sexually assaulted or abused at any age.

Difficulties in your second chakra can develop early in your life as you learn to walk and talk and start exploring the world through your senses. Problems in this chakra show up in the reproductive organs and also in the abdomen. Diseases and health issues often associated with the second chakra include problems with the male and female reproductive organs, sexual dysfunction, inflammatory bowel disease, appendicitis, chronic low back or sciatic nerve pain, and bladder or urinary problems.

Archetypes

The martyr and the monarch are the archetypes of the second chakra. The monarch enjoys abundance and is happy, while the martyr sacrifices and suffers. Unlike the first chakra victim, the martyr does hold herself responsible but isn't empowered because she doesn't have a great enough sense of self and therefore feels helpless to change anything. Martyrs devote themselves to making sure

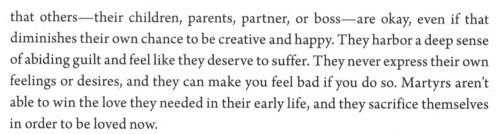

that others—their children, parents, partner, or boss—are okay, even if that diminishes their own chance to be creative and happy. They harbor a deep sense of abiding guilt and feel like they deserve to suffer. They never express their own feelings or desires, and they can make you feel bad if you do so. Martyrs aren't able to win the love they needed in their early life, and they sacrifice themselves in order to be loved now.

Monarchs, on the other hand, feel good about themselves. They trust their body and understand what they hunger for, but they know when they've reached their limit and don't overly indulge or become addicted to anything. This positive archetype represents not only earthly pleasure but also power in the world. Monarchs surround themselves with beauty, and they enjoy the fullness of life; they are open to others and comfortable in their home. Their inner life may not be very well developed, but they are happy with their material possessions.

Spiritual Aspects

The *bija* mantra for the second chakra is *Vam*, and when you repeat this seed sound near a body of water, it strengthens the fluids in the body to circulate better. From Hindu mythology comes a sea creature called the *makara*, somewhat like a crocodile, that is the carrier for the seed sound. The makara represents your animal instincts—the passions and desires that lurk in the watery depths of your unconscious and have to be harnessed. The gods and goddesses are known for the dangerous creatures they use as their vehicles to show they have tamed their dark inner forces, like the great goddess Durga, who is seen riding a lion.

The ruler of the second chakra is Vishnu, who is the lord of preservation. He is the fulcrum holding the life-giving balance between Brahma, the force of creation in the first chakra, and Shiva, the force of destruction in the third. He does this by incarnating in different periods of time on earth in order to restore balance. He incarnated as Lord Rama to bring righteousness to earth, and most recently as Lord Krishna, the "divine lover" whose task was to bring an infusion of love.

In the astrological realm, the second chakra is associated with the moon. As the moon waxes and wanes, it influences your emotions, your body, and in women, their menstrual cycles. The second chakra is also associated with the planet Pluto, which represents your ability to transform. These two heavenly bodies influence the second chakra as the energy center of pleasure, intimacy, feeling and sensation, change, and movement.

Know When to Give Your Second Chakra a Tune-Up

The second chakra is connected to the ovaries in women and the testes in men. If your chakras aren't well-balanced, you may develop problems with the related gland or organ. Getting diagnosed with cervical cancer at a young age meant my second chakra, as well as my first, had probably been in distress for a while. If you're dealing with sexual problems, recurrent STDs, fertility issues, or impotence, you will want to examine your second chakra issues and find the underlying emotional cause, as well as get traditional medical help.

To check your second chakra, honestly answer the following questions:

- Are you generally pessimistic, and do you say things such as: "I'm never going to find a life partner" or "I can't lose weight" or "I can't earn enough money?"

- Are you unable to both give and receive pleasure?

- Are you unable to both give and receive money?

- Do you have a crushing sense of somehow failing in life?

- Have you ignored your ethics in exchange for money, power, or sex?

- Do you care too much about what others think of you?

- Do you put aside your own dreams?

- Do you frequently feel like you're all alone in the world?

- Are you unable to release what has happened in the past? Are you still plotting your revenge?

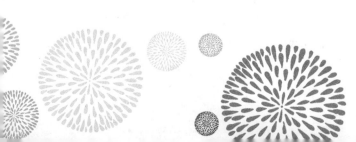 Do you always feel the need to buck authority?

If you answered yes to three or more of these questions, chances are your second chakra could use a tune-up.

How to Clear Second Chakra Blockages

Some simple ways of clearing this chakra are finding a hobby or activity you enjoy that allows you to express your creativity and surround yourself with beauty—art; music; flowers, especially roses, irises, and sweet-smelling blooms; water bodywork like Watsu (water shiatsu); essential oils of musk or sandalwood; and affirmations that banish guilt like *I enjoy my life and all its pleasures, and I let my feelings move through me in a graceful, flowing way*. I took up riding horses to help open and expand my second chakra.

Touch is vitally important for healing your second chakra and for your health in general. A hug, a massage, holding your pet—any type of gentle touch takes you into harmonious relationship with others. Without touch, you are "out of touch" with yourself and everyone else.

To keep this chakra up and running, you can work with the color orange, a warm and positive color that symbolizes second chakra energy. It integrates the red from the first chakra with the yellow wisdom from the third chakra. You can also wear or decorate with the color orange. The stones that work with the second chakra are amber, carnelian, and fire opal, and the metal is gold. Incenses that enhance this center are gardenia and orris root. Since this chakra is connected to the element of water, remember to stay hydrated. Find water bottled in glass that still has its natural minerals, and drink freely and often.

THE THIRD AND FOURTH CHAKRAS

The third and fourth energy centers pack a big punch. The third chakra is the furnace that generates the energy to make the leap into the fourth chakra, the heart. The heart is the center point of your basic seven chakras, the point of balance between the lower three physical chakras and the upper three spiritual chakras.

The Third Chakra—Power

The life force of energy healers is the power that resides at their core. It's the fire that ignites your internal engines to power up and heal someone in need. It's also the power that charges up faith in yourself to get the job done. I'm talking about the third chakra—your power center.

The third chakra, also known as the solar plexus chakra, is located halfway between your navel and sternum, and is a lustrous yellow. If you're constantly living in your head, expending lots of mental energy, yours will be a more intense yellow. The third chakra is all about your mental clarity, the focal point of your mental field. It's your sense of self and your power center. Your authenticity lives in this chakra. In Sanskrit, the third chakra is called *manipura*, which means "lustrous gem."

The element most closely associated with the third chakra is fire. Fire is transformative—it burns wood to turn it into heat; it heats water and turns it into steam; it turns a candle into a source of light. Therefore, the governing principle of the third chakra is transformation. The elements of the first and second chakras—earth and water—move downward, while the element of fire goes upward, reaching to higher levels. The third chakra is thus the internal combustion machine that can generate the power for you to cross the chasm and reach the heart chakra. The fire of this chakra allows you to release dysfunctional thoughts and old behavior patterns. If you are solidly grounded and your emotions are flowing easily through you, then the fire of your third chakra can power up your will and convert it into action. When fire burns, it produces light. The sense that can pick up the light is sight, and the sense organs connected to this chakra are the eyes.

The Third Chakra's Biggest Obstacle

Problems can start to manifest in this solar plexus chakra between eighteen months and four years old. This is the time you develop your first definition of self and begin to learn impulse control. Self-control translates into pride and self-worth, while any type of abuse at this stage of life can create a sense of shame. Shame can render you powerless and block your energy by making you feel unworthy and inferior. It can stop you from being your true, authentic self and can cause you to run from the truth. It can hinder your individuality.

Shame stems from your perception of how you're doing in your own eyes or in the eyes of others. Your parents may have constantly said, "You ought to be ashamed of yourself!" Maybe you were called names or labeled as lazy, stupid, or homely. Shame is always being aware of your personal defects. When there is a voice in your head that keeps saying, "I never do anything right," or "I'll never be good (or strong, sexy, thin, and so on) enough," or "I'll never get a promotion," you are probably dealing with shame, which can hold you back from realizing your true potential.

The Health of Your Third Chakra

Your solar plexus chakra fires up your strength of will and fortifies your personal power. When you own the power that this chakra is generating, then you know your own worth and can fully embrace your own life story. You use your willpower to empower yourself in all aspects of life. Plus, you begin to gain a keen awareness, have heightened intelligence, and take control of all the challenges that come your way.

When the third chakra is running on full steam, you have taken control. You have assumed responsibility for whatever you need to handle. You take back any power you handed over to others. You seek the best ways to heal rather than bowing to what others say. You are willing to leave a job or career if it doesn't feel right and find whatever it is in life that will allow you to be the person you want to be.

Issues concerning your personal power and authentic self are most likely to cause problems with your third chakra. For example, if you were teased and bullied as a child, or if you lived with controlling parents, you may have experienced, or still experience, problems with this chakra. As an adult, having low self-esteem or living with an excessively dominating partner or staying in a marriage or job that isn't working for you may cause problems in your third chakra.

The third chakra holds the most organs of all the chakras, and these organs play a part in digestion. Problems in this chakra typically show up in the liver, gallbladder, stomach, spleen, pancreas, or kidneys. Diseases and health concerns commonly associated with the third chakra include illnesses involving the pancreas (most notably diabetes and hypoglycemia), digestive difficulties, liver disease, hiatal hernias, gallstones, hemorrhoids, varicose veins, and problems with the spleen.

Archetypes

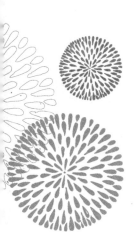

The solar plexus chakra's dysfunctional archetype is the servant, who is not aware of her own worth. The victim archetype of the first chakra victim and the martyr archetype of the second chakra are more negative than that of the servant, but servants don't take responsibility for their own self-esteem, instead relying on others for acknowledgment. Their lack of self-confidence often leaves servants hidden in the background, and without strong boundaries, they easily fall to manipulation by others. In this way, an abused child then becomes a battered wife who believes she deserves her husband's punishment. An authoritarian father's son never develops a strong will and may wind up never getting his work acknowledged.

The third chakra generates a lot of power, and when you recognize that power as your own, you are the hero of your own story and exemplify the positive third chakra archetype of the warrior. The warrior is the strongest of all the archetypes because warriors know how to use their willpower to empower themselves in life. They are able to face any challenges head-on instead of running from them. Learning that you are indeed responsible for your own life is one of the greatest challenges. You have to take back your power from others, whether that means choosing a career your parents don't approve of, standing up to a bully, or leaving a bad relationship. The warrior in you can do that when you are in sync with your third chakra power. However much warriors can achieve their goals and thrive, they don't yet understand that we are all one in the spiritual realm.

Spiritual Aspects

The seed sound of the third chakra is *Ram*. When repeated, it bolsters the digestive fire. Fire moves in an upward direction, so repetition of this mantra directs the kundalini energy up the chakras. The vehicle of Agni, the fire god, is the ram that carries the seed sound. A ram is a strong animal that meets its foes head-on; in "olden days," the ram's horn was used in battle to blast the sound of courage to the soldiers.

Rudra, the presiding deity of the third chakra, is the wrathful form of Shiva. His job is to destroy one cycle of creation so the next can be born. It is the fierce fire of your will that creates enough movement for your energy to rise through the chakras toward the goal of higher consciousness. It is the fire of your will that can make you face your challenges, take action, and move toward a new goal.

In astrological terms, the sun is the ruling planet of this energy center. Just as we received our nourishment through the umbilical cord when our navel was our source of life, the bright yellow sun is the radiant source of life for those of us on planet Earth. The navel area is the cauldron for the fire of the third chakra, supplying you with vital energy. The planet Mars is the warrior planet and is thus also associated with the solar plexus chakra.

Know When to Give Your Third Chakra a Tune-Up

The controlling gland of the third chakra is the pancreas, which regulates blood sugar and also processes your emotions. The metabolic fire of this chakra turns nutrients into energy. If there is not enough energy produced, there can be problems in some aspect of digestion or hypoglycemia. On the other hand, diabetes, hyperglycemia, and ulcers come from excess energy. You can actually be both deficient and excessive, swinging back and forth between high and low blood sugar. When I was young, I felt like I was on that roller-coaster ride. A Chinese medical doctor would say this is a deficiency of both yin (negative) and yang (positive) energy and would treat both at the same time.

In dealing with an unbalanced third chakra, you might find that you have a hard time expressing your emotions. You may hide your true feelings because you're afraid there may be repercussions, such as people won't like you anymore. You might hear yourself saying, "I don't get enough approval" or "I don't feel safe." To check your solar plexus, honestly answer these questions:

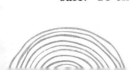

- Do you have a lot of suppressed anger, fear, or grief?

- Do you hold on to your resentments?

- Do you tend to blame others for your problems?

- Are you jealous of others? Do you think the grass is greener somewhere else?

- Do you feel like you never have enough time?

- Are you a control freak?

- Do you worry that others will overpower you?

- Do you have to win?

- Do you feel good about yourself only when you receive outside approval?

- Do you often stand with your arms crossed in front of your chest?

If you answered yes to three or more of these questions, chances are your third chakra could use a tune-up.

How to Clear Third Chakra Blockages

How do you balance your third chakra? You need to make your personal power your top priority. No more putting aside who you really are and what you really want to do. The time for you to take center stage is *now*!

Since the *solar* plexus chakra is related to the fire element, being outside in the sun is good but only in the early morning or as it is beginning to set so you don't get too hot. Connecting to the earth and the sun is very healing for the third chakra. Do something physical outdoors—a little stretching, walking, swimming, or gardening. Taking a walk by the ocean or any other body of water is also healing.

To really open your third chakra and clear out blockages, you can start by becoming more aware of your actions and doing selfless service. Any act of courage—doing what's right, not what pleases everyone else—strengthens this chakra.

To give a boost to your third chakra, use the incense or essential oils of cinnamon, sandalwood, musk, or ginger. Yellow stones such as amber, golden topaz, yellow citrine, tiger's eye, or rutilated quartz are good for bringing this powerful chakra into balance. Ultimately, having a balanced third chakra means that you accept personal responsibility, self-discipline, confidence, and energy. You also take risks but will always have a little time for fun!

Third Chakra Exercise: Looking in the Mirror

If you feel like your third chakra needs a shot in the arm, try this: Stand in front of a full-length mirror and take some time to really look at yourself. Don't judge what you see! Don't fret over certain body parts—those thighs, that belly, or what used to be a neck. Look at yourself in the mirror with compassion and love. As you're looking in the mirror, name five of your best qualities; say them out loud. Remind yourself of the things you most like about you. Sincerely say the following affirmations out loud: *I deserve love. I deserve respect. I am enough. I love myself.* Keep looking at yourself as you say these words. How does it feel? Do you believe what you are saying? Do it until you actually feel the truth of those words.

The Fourth Chakra—Balance

An open heart chakra is the hallmark of an energy healer. Energy healers are often motivated by compassion and love to help all of humanity. You, too, are on your way to becoming an energy healer. You can tap into your heartfelt love and compassion right here as you learn about your fourth chakra, the heart chakra.

The fourth chakra is the color of lush green grass. It's the easiest chakra to connect to, the one you can feel the most easily. It's all about loving yourself just the way you are, not when you're twenty pounds thinner or you've found the right soul mate or you've landed the job of your dreams.

The fourth chakra is where you come home to your heart, the very center of the chakra system. The main function of the first three chakras is to connect you to the world, while the fourth chakra's duty is to form the link, or bridge, between the three physical chakras below it and the three spiritual chakras above it. In other words, this chakra bridges the lower and upper worlds, bringing body and spirit into balance. From here, you are given the opportunity to reach out and touch both heaven and earth. That's why touch is the sense related to the heart chakra.

In Sanskrit, the name of this chakra is *anahata*, which means "unhurt," "unstruck," or "unbeaten." The governing principle of this chakra is equilibrium. It's all about balance—coming into balance within yourself as well as with your relationships and whatever is happening in your environment.

The heart chakra is associated with the element of air. You have now leaped from earth, water, and fire into the air in its purest form—without color, form, fragrance, or taste. Air moves in all directions, circulating oxygen and bringing it into the breath, the vital energy needed to live. With all of this clear, clean, healthy, and fresh air comes more space and clarity. So when your fourth chakra is balanced, you have the spaciousness to be more contemplative and more conscious. You also have more clarity and breathing room to be aware of your needs and those of others. Being more conscious helps you connect with your inner self. That's why self-care is so important in this chakra; it helps you reach this state of inner balance.

When you're connected with your inner self, you begin to love yourself more, which helps you reach out to others. You have to love yourself before you can really love someone else, which requires an acceptance of humanity in all its dual aspects: body and mind, light and shadow, child and adult, giver and taker, good and evil. Self-love implies the ability to listen and respond to your own needs as well as to the needs of others.

The heart chakra develops between four and seven years of age, when you are establishing relationships with your peers and family, and creating the persona of who you are.

The Fourth Chakra's Biggest Obstacle

Your emotions power your chakras, literally. When you're in a state of love, your heart will be open and tapping into the energy of the environment. Then when someone says something unkind to you, your heart closes because you can't bear the pain. The fourth chakra's biggest obstacle just showed up—heartbreak. Heartbreak can shatter your heart in a thousand ways. There are certain life situations that can wreak havoc on your fourth chakra, such as rejection, emotional or physical neglect and abuse, chronic depression, codependency, the betrayal of a cheating partner, or loss (as in the death of a loved one or the dissolution of a relationship). Any of these can cause you to live with fear of heartbreak, which will cause your heart chakra to close.

The Health of Your Fourth Chakra

Giving and receiving love is the central function of the heart chakra. You don't want a heart that's closed. You won't feel the pain, but you won't be able to feel any joy either. And the bad news is that it affects your entire body. If your heart is closed, your blood pressure could go up; your cardiovascular system can become compromised. When your fourth chakra is healthy, you can fully love and accept yourself as you are. You can live from a place of love for all of humanity and for all life forms on the planet. You feel worthy to receive love. You take responsibility for keeping your heart open, for forgiving others and yourself.

Located in the center of the chest, the fourth chakra rules over the lungs, thymus (the governing gland for this chakra), upper back, ribs, arms, and hands. This energy center rules the heart—the central, life-giving organ in the body.

Typical fourth chakra diseases and health concerns include problems with the heart, such as congestive heart failure, heart attack, or chest pain (angina); difficulties with circulation; disorders of the lungs, including pneumonia, lung cancer, bronchitis, and emphysema; breast cancer and disorders of the breast, like cysts or mastitis; shoulder, arm, and hand issues, such as carpal tunnel and tension or pain between the shoulder blades; immune system deficiencies (this shows up in the first chakra too); asthma; and all kinds of allergies.

Archetypes

The performer is the dysfunctional archetype of the fourth chakra—these are people who hide their dark side while playing at love. Performers make it look like everything is fine but cannot accept the responsibility that comes with real intimacy. When someone starts getting too close, performers protect themselves by damaging the relationship in some way. Their vulnerability cannot be exposed, so they are closed off from loving and being loved. Performers can be very skilled at seduction while still protecting against being wounded by not loving the person who's been seduced. It's classic codependency: resisting love while, at the same time, blaming their partner for anything that goes wrong.

The lover is, naturally, the positive archetype for the heart chakra. Lovers love all of humanity and all life forms on the planet as well as themselves. They understand the importance of forgiving others and themselves. They feel worthy of receiving love, and they allow it to flow through their open heart chakra and expand in all directions. This is why everyone loves a lover.

Spiritual Aspects

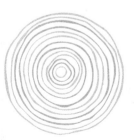

In many spiritual traditions, the heart is considered the residence of God, the temple of the Higher Self. In the tradition of Judaic Kabbalah, the center of the Tree of Life is associated with the heart; in the Christian Kabbalah, it is represented by the Sacred Heart of Jesus, the Christ; in traditional Chinese medicine, the heart is home to *Shen*, or Spirit, within each person, called the Emperor or Sovereign

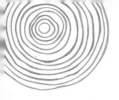

Ruler. The great wizard Merlin called the heart the "gateway between worlds." In shamanic traditions, the heart is the Keeper of Wisdom, inner truth. And living from the heart is what the Ascended Masters teach about enlightenment.

The bija mantra for the fourth chakra is *Yam*, the seed sound that vibrates the spiritual heart and releases blockages in that area. The black antelope or musk deer is the carrier of the sound. An antelope leaps with joy but can also be caught in illusion. And just as we hold within ourselves cosmic consciousness yet search for it outside of ourselves, the musk deer runs around searching for the enchanting smell of musk, not knowing that the wonderful odor comes from itself.

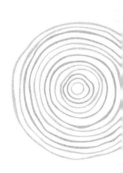

Ishana Rudra Shiva is the Hindu deity presiding over the fourth chakra. He is detached from the world, peaceful and beneficent. He allows the holy Ganges River, the divine stream of knowledge of the self, to flow through his hair so the force of its mighty waters will be softened as the river falls from heaven to earth. He symbolizes the way to live in harmony inside and out, in both the upper and lower worlds.

Astrologically, the planet Venus, named after the Roman goddess of love and beauty, is naturally associated with the heart chakra. (She's called Aphrodite in Greek mythology.) How you approach love relationships can be influenced by where Venus is on your astrological chart. For example, if Venus is in Cancer, you would more likely be concerned about how secure your relationship is, but if Venus is in Aries, it would be the thrill of the conquest that most excites you.

Know When to Give Your Fourth Chakra a Tune-Up

Often, what happens when you've been emotionally shattered is that you build a wall around your heart and lock your pain inside. There are ways to remove the wall and express this pain; you can talk about your grief, write about your feelings in your journal, sweat out your feelings with exercise, or do anything you can to move this negative energy out of your body.

It took me years to reverse the damaging pattern of protecting my heart, which had collapsed inside my rib cage when I was a child. I didn't have a safe space to

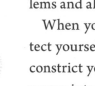

express love or my feelings in a direct way, so I was plagued with immune problems and allergies.

When you close off your heart, you feel helpless. Sometimes you try to protect yourself after a painful breakup by becoming emotionally cold. When you constrict your energy flow and close yourself off, you stop the flow of love that moves into you and out to others. To check your heart chakra, honestly answer these questions:

- Is love scary to you?

- Do you give and receive love easily?

- Have you ever felt betrayed or rejected?

- Are you unable to forgive yourself and others for past mistakes?

- Are you overly critical or judgmental of others?

- Do you need to develop the higher attributes, such as altruism, compassion, forgiveness, hope, trust, or harmony?

- Have you been diagnosed with heart-related problems, lung or breast disease, or pneumonia?

- Do your hands or arms ache?

If you answered yes to three or more of these questions, chances are your fourth chakra could use a tune-up.

How to Clear Fourth Chakra Blockages

When you're in the clutches of grief or resentment, it's hard to open your heart and feel the pain. But that's what an energy healer can help you do. Open up. Face your fears. Cry a thousand tears if you have to, but don't close your heart. If you do, it won't just prevent heartache—it will also prevent any love from flowing in or out.

One way to get through grief is through breath work, in which you use the key element of air to reconnect you to your heart, thus allowing your positive energy to flow again. Once you have removed the blockage, you can put the hurt you've experienced to work by becoming more compassionate to the suffering of others, perhaps even choosing to be an energy healer. Wounded healers who have worked through their wounds, without hiding or burying them, are uniquely prepared to help others.

Another great way to open your heart and clear any blockages is by caring for a pet. A dog, cat, horse (my personal favorite), and even a bird can teach you how to open your heart. Pets love you unconditionally and make it all right for you to love again.

To keep the energy flowing in your fourth chakra, you can also set an intention to love and care for yourself. Chances are you don't spend enough time really appreciating who you are. Go ahead and appreciate your uniqueness, your inner beauty, your courage, and your kindness—all of your finest qualities. Meditation and journaling help you dig out of the pit where you buried any hope of experiencing real love and bring down the brick wall surrounding your heart.

To help open your heart chakra, try incense or essential oils of lavender, jasmine, yarrow, marjoram, or meadowsweet. Use green stones such as emerald, green tourmaline, malachite, or green jade. Pink stones, like rose quartz, are also associated with love and the heart chakra. In the Chinese medicine system vegetables—especially green ones—help with balance, as they are neither yin nor yang.

When your energy is freely flowing through your heart chakra—connecting mind and body, inner and outer self—you'll feel a profound sense of peace and fulfillment that will prepare you for your higher chakras. Now let's head further up into the spiritual fifth and sixth chakras.

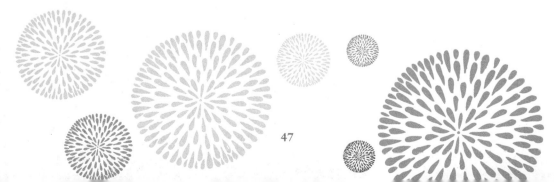

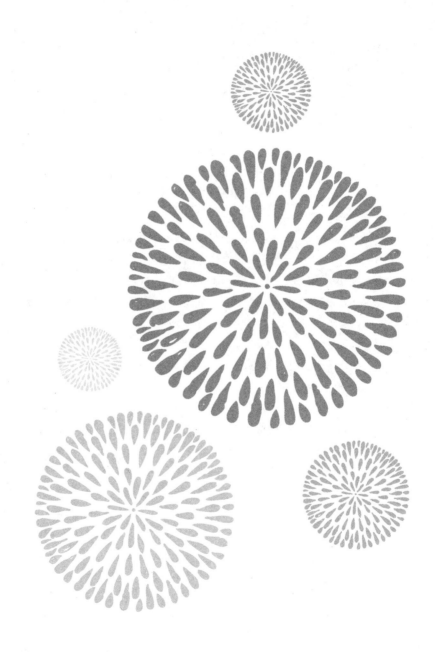

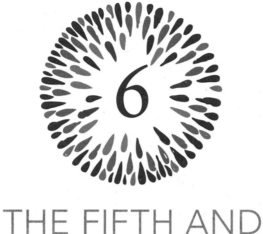

THE FIFTH AND
SIXTH CHAKRAS

You have just learned about the lower three chakras that ground you on the earth as well as the fourth chakra that bridges the ascent to the higher spiritual energy centers. Now it's time to unlock the upper energy centers, where your spiritual powers begin to reveal themselves on the continuing journey to your mastery of energy healing.

The Fifth Chakra—Expression

The fifth chakra is located in the center of the throat, and it connects the feelings in your heart center with the thoughts in your brow chakra, allowing you to express your emotions and thoughts. Being the first of the spiritual chakras, the fifth chakra is the portal through which you bring spirit into the physical realm, where you connect with your true essence. In Sanskrit, the fifth chakra is called *vishuddha*, which means "purification"—purity in expressing how you feel and what you want, and releasing any tendency to bury your truth.

This chakra's main task is communication. Here you give voice to your unique expression of spirit—your creativity. The cobalt-blue fifth chakra, or throat chakra, is where you get to express what you have created. Remember, your creativity was born in the second chakra. The fifth chakra is the place where the creativity of the second chakra manifests. Here's where you rely on your inner voice and the truth. This is where you have to really listen carefully so you can hear the beat that will lead you to your true calling.

The governing principle of this chakra is resonance. Resonance means that vibrations of similar frequency are joined with each other in rhythm. The element associated with the throat chakra is ether or sound, which is produced by the rhythmic vibration of molecules of air. You give off a vibration that is the culmination of the activity that has occurred in all the previous four chakras. In other words, you experience the inner workings of those four chakras simply as an overall quality of vibration. When you meet someone, you register this person as a vibration. The higher the vibration, the more harmonious that person is.

This chakra is vital because it helps you tune into the vibe of the world. When a person, an idea, a particular setting, or a piece of music resonates with you, you experience that person, thing, or place with greater joy, energy, and clarity, and you want to spend more time there. When you hear something that rings true for you, you experience more harmony in your inner world, an expansive quality that then goes out to the world. So if you want to help change the world for the better, spend more time in meditation. This raises your vibration, and your vibration emanates out into the world, where it will help raise the vibrations of others. The more people vibrating at a higher frequency, the more quickly *everyone's* vibration will go higher and the better the world will be. That's what healing circles, which we'll talk about at the end of this book, are all about.

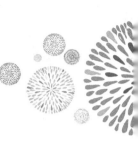

The throat chakra is also the place where you can access that quiet, wise inner voice that will guide you in any situation—assuming, of course, that you listen to it!

The Fifth Chakra's Biggest Obstacle

Problems can develop in your throat chakra between the ages of about seven and twelve, when you learn symbolic thinking and develop communication skills. Trouble happens at any age when you're not allowed to express your true feelings—the biggest obstacle standing in the way of a clear functioning fifth chakra. Before you can resonate with others, you need to resonate within yourself, which means living your truth.

Truth is the underlying energy that powers the fifth chakra. And this includes being true to yourself in how you live and what you take in on a daily basis. As a society, we are constantly being bombarded with every possible message: advertising and marketing try to sell us products we don't need, "reality" television shows use scripts to lure us into the drama, news stations try to instill fear in us by focusing on violence, and T-shirts proclaim negative and hurtful slogans. Amidst all of this manipulation, it's imperative to see through to *your* truth.

The Health of Your Fifth Chakra

Living your truth is the key to the health of the fifth chakra. *Speaking your truth* means expressing who you are—your feelings, thoughts, beliefs—through speaking, writing, singing, or other artistic creations or through your work, your hobbies, the way you decorate your house, even the clothes you wear. If your fifth chakra is in balance, creativity flows and communication rocks. You are living with integrity according to your dreams and visions, loving who you are, and appreciating the blessings in your life. Living your truth is a daily practice of checking in with yourself, listening to your inner guidance, and observing your interactions with the world to see if you are resonating with higher Source.

When this chakra is healthy, you take responsibility for expressing how you feel and what you want in life. You deliver your messages clearly and respect

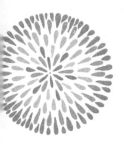

those who receive them. You speak from the heart and don't lie. People trust you because you back up your words with positive action. You are trusted—you say what you mean and mean what you say because you know the importance and power of your word.

Throat chakra issues are concerned with speaking your truth and expressing your creativity and true emotions. Some classic life situations that can negatively affect your fifth chakra include dealing with controlling or abusive parents, partners, or bosses; listening to excessive conversation or gossip; being extremely fearful of speaking in groups or in public; and bottling up anger and frustration until you almost explode.

The fifth chakra rules over the thyroid and parathyroid glands. Problems in this chakra typically show up in the shoulders, throat, neck, ears, mouth, jaw, teeth, vocal chords, nasal sinuses, cervical vertebrae, trachea, and esophagus. Common fifth chakra diseases and health concerns include disorders of the voice, mouth, teeth, or gums; tight neck and other neck problems; stiff shoulders; swollen glands in your throat or recurrent sore throats; throat cancer; chronic childhood tonsillitis; chronic sinus problems; TMJ; and hypo- or hyperthyroidism, thyroid cancer, Hashimoto's or Graves' diseases.

Archetypes

The silent child is the dysfunctional archetype for the fifth chakra. The silent child feels safest when silent and has a hard time expressing anger and frustration. The silent child blocks or suppresses scary or painful feelings; heaven knows, in the silent child's mind, if you told people what you really think or feel, they might leave you! If you are a silent child, you might feel like no one loves you or listens to you. That's the problem with swallowing your shame and guilt; it also swallows your potential for vitality and joy in life.

The broadcaster, the positive fifth chakra archetype, can express her feelings and her desires in life by speaking out, even in emails and texts. Broadcasters can also deliver their message nonverbally through art, music, and dance. Broadcasters know how important and powerful the spoken word is and that

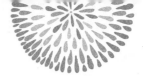

gossip and verbal criticism are not from the Higher Self. They deliver their messages clearly, respect the recipients, and follow their words up with right action. Broadcasters don't lie, and they speak from the heart, so you know you can trust them.

Spiritual Aspects

The fifth chakra is all about purity in how you express your feelings and desires, and about the ability to speak your truth instead of burying it. The deity of the throat chakra is Panchavaktra Shiva, who has five heads representing the five senses and the corresponding five elements: smell/earth, taste/water, sight/fire, touch/air, and sound/space. Shiva plays the *damaru*, a drum that makes fourteen different sounds that are said to be the source of the Sanskrit language. The drum produces overtones that create the primal sound of *Aum*.

The seed sound for this chakra is *Ham*. When it is pronounced correctly, repetition of this bija syllable makes your voice sound sweet because of the cerebrospinal fluid that is released into the throat. The elephant, with its enormous ears and graceful stride, shows the importance of rhythm and sound and is the carrier of this seed sound.

Astrologically, the fifth chakra is associated with the planets Jupiter and Mercury. Jupiter is known as the *guru* in Sanskrit, the dispeller of darkness, while Mercury is the planet of communication. As the winged Roman messenger of the gods, Mercury can influence how you think, create, and express yourself. Speaking, writing, online communication, and books are within Mercury's domain—which is why communication goes topsy-turvy when Mercury goes retrograde!

Know When to Give Your Fifth Chakra a Tune-Up

What do you do when you can't express your feelings or thoughts? Perhaps you reach for your favorite comfort food instead of dealing with a confrontation. You might even be fearful that if you tell the truth, there will be harmful consequences. Historically women have been taught to keep their thoughts and

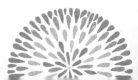

feelings to themselves. Then there is that old adage "Children are meant to be seen and not heard." And what about those who can't express their true sexual orientation or gender without fear of reprisal?

When you ignore or hide your feelings and when you feel like you can't express yourself, you are preventing your energy from flowing freely in this chakra, and ultimately, it will shut down. You may also have other difficulties with communication in this chakra, such as stuttering or fear of speaking. For many years, I was so scared of public speaking that I would rather have been in the coffin than giving the eulogy! You might also feel like you've lost the rhythm of life, have trouble taking in what others are saying, or suffer excessive shyness. To check your throat chakra, honestly answer these questions:

- Are you unable to ask for what you need?

- Are you always self-editing what you say?

- Do you frequently bite your tongue and fail to speak your mind?

- Are you unable to act on inner guidance?

- Do you have a weak sense of timing and rhythm?

- Are you chronically hoarse?

- Are you honest with yourself?

- Do you have chronic sore throats or sinus problems?

- Do you often experience pain in your neck, cervical vertebrae, or shoulders?

- Do you talk too much or too loudly or stutter, or are you reluctant to speak?

- Are you tone deaf?

- Are you overly shy?

If you answered yes to three or more of these questions, chances are your fifth chakra could use a tune-up.

How to Clear Fifth Chakra Blockages

To get more in touch with your true self that wants to be heard, I strongly suggest journaling. Get an empty journal and write in it daily or even hourly. Or get a phone app and put your notes there. (When I was a lawyer, I constantly jotted down my feelings in the margins of my trial notes.) Your notes can be as brief as one letter; for example, *J* can stand for jealous and *F* for fearful. Your notes can safely hold all your thoughts, feelings, and insights—a powerful way to begin expressing your truth. Once you trust yourself to be honest in your notes, you will begin to trust that you can be honest in the world. If your relationship needs help, try couples therapy to improve communication. A wonderful way to open your throat is by taking singing lessons or participating in a choir or singing group.

Fruit is one of the best types of sustenance for supporting the fifth chakra. This is because fruit is lowest on the food chain, simply dropping to the ground when ripe. It is the quickest of all solid foods to pass through your system, leaving your energy free to head up to your higher chakras.

Since this chakra is a magnificent cobalt-blue color, you can introduce blue stones, including turquoise, aquamarine, or blue sapphire. Fragrances or incense that enhance this chakra include frankincense, mace, rose, and jasmine. The rewards of balancing this energy center are more powerful communication, greater creativity, and ease and flow to life.

The Sixth Chakra—Intuition

The sixth chakra, called the brow chakra or the third eye, is where your master mind plugs into a new type of wisdom from beyond this realm, providing amazing insights that will allow you to solve any problem. The sixth chakra is

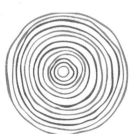

located just above your eyebrows in the center of your forehead. Because the sixth chakra is located in your head rather than in your torso like the first five chakras, it has a slightly different nature and is the control center for some very powerful gifts: thinking, wisdom, psychic gifts, and intuition. It's a stunning indigo color, which indicates peace and tranquility. It's all about your intuition, your ability to plan, forecast, sense, and know.

In the previous chakra, information came to you in the form of vibrations or sound and through symbols like words. Here, you get data through images. The governing principle, then, of the sixth chakra is image formation. You create or receive information visually on the internal screen of your mind and then interpret and store it; this includes what you see, what you imagine, and what you perceive through psychic and intuitive channels.

The brow chakra is called the *ajna* in Sanskrit, meaning both "to perceive" and "to command." This chakra is the center of both conscious and subconscious beliefs, and it provides a window into a reality beyond this one, allowing you to receive information beyond your basic five senses. This is where you can gain entry into the unified energy field through your intuitive abilities.

The gifts that may become available when you expand this chakra include telepathy (inner communication of thoughts), precognition (information about the future), remote viewing (seeing distant locations), and clairvoyance (visual insight). The governing gland of the chakra is the pineal, which is in the center of your head close to your eyes. Known as the seat of the soul, the pineal gland uses light fluctuations to produce various hormones that control more than one hundred bodily functions.

The Sixth Chakra's Biggest Obstacle

Problems commonly develop in the brow chakra at the high school and college ages when hormones are at their highest and you are learning to hear your intuitive voice. As an adult, if your mind is overstimulated and full of anxiety and

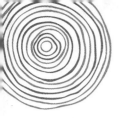

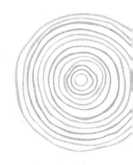

worry, your intuitive voice can get muffled or silenced. Overthinking is therefore the biggest obstacle to sixth chakra health. Overthinking can cut off access to your inner voice and preoccupy you with highly irrational left-brain fears and emotions. By rationalizing and theorizing, you can stay stuck in the realm of the mind while your vital energy stagnates. Not only that, but you can lose out on the creativity, intuition, and wisdom that is available when your sixth chakra is in balance. To ward off this obstacle, reconnect with the element of earth, develop warm personal relationships, and learn to take pleasure in your body.

The Health of Your Sixth Chakra

When this center is balanced, your left brain is clear and focused and works in conjunction with your open and intuitive right brain. This gives you immediate access to your deepest wisdom. You also have the gift of inner sight, and you trust your inner guidance. Living from that place of deep trust means you live impeccably and love all of life. As someone who can interpret metaphors and symbols that come from your intuitive voice, you will be talented in any of the healing arts because you are in sync with your inner core.

Intuitive guidance often comes in your dreams, which combine memories with your imagination. Through symbolic visual images, your dreams give your psyche a way to communicate, telling you what's going on in your unconscious. Each element in a dream is vital, so take the time to write your dreams down so you won't forget them.

The key sixth chakra issue is being in tune with your sixth sense, your intuitive power. Some typical life situations that can disturb this chakra include: people in your life who put you down or discount your intuition, as well as pessimistic or negative people in your space. Signs of a flagging sixth chakra are poor memory, poor concentration, nightmares or hallucinations, and paranoia.

This energy center rules over the eyes, nose, brain, and neurological system. It is associated with the pineal gland, which in turn affects all the other endocrine glands and creates a link between the brain and the immune system. It also affects how trauma is registered in your brain. When this area is out of balance, the following sixth chakra diseases and health concerns can happen: eye problems, such as poor eyesight, glaucoma, cataracts, macular degeneration, and blindness; conditions of the upper or frontal sinuses; headaches; stroke; neurological disturbances; and brain tumors.

Archetypes

The thinker is the dysfunctional archetype of the sixth chakra. Thinkers try to live from the rationality of the left brain and believe that emotions are highly irrational, so they rarely confront their feelings and fears. Thinkers have an overstimulated mind, making them anxious from too much thinking and worrying. This cuts off access to the inner voice. Thinkers may develop highly opinionated ideas based on inadequate facts instead of relying on their life experience, creativity, intuition, and the inner wisdom that comes from a balanced sixth chakra. Thinkers are helped by reconnecting to the earth, having warm personal relationships, and learning to appreciate their physical body.

The seer is the positive sixth chakra archetype. In Native traditions, the seer was usually an elder of the tribe, respected for deep inner wisdom. When our seniors are not respected or honored, we have no wise elder to go to for help. A true seer is gifted with inner sight, has learned to trust inner guidance, and lives impeccably, loving all life. Seers can be skilled in any field because they are in touch with their inner core and can understand metaphors and symbols.

Spiritual Aspects

For the third eye chakra, the seed sound is *Om*, the primal sound of the cosmos that holds within it the consciousness of unity. The deity presiding over this chakra is Shiva-Shakti: Shiva is the solar male on the right side, and Shakti is the lunar female on the left. This half-male, half-female god-goddess symbolizes the merger of pure consciousness and energy, showing that there is only One. There is no more duality, just as the third eye sees the past, present, and future as one. In states of deep meditation, you can experience the *soma* (nectar) that fills you with bliss. When advanced yogis absorb this soma, they unlock the key to immortality.

Astrologically, the planet Neptune rules the sixth chakra. Neptune is the planet farthest from the sun. Named for the Roman ruler of the sea, Neptune is as deep and mysterious as the depths of the ocean. It is considered a visionary planet and thus influences your ability to create. It is also called the planet of illusion, and in this way can lead to self-destructive fantasies. One of the big obstacles to balancing and clearing the sixth chakra is getting stuck in illusion. When you think you know how things should be, when you are attached to a particular perspective, you are not seeing with any real clarity, like an anorexic looking in the mirror and believing she is fat.

Know When to Give Your Sixth Chakra a Tune-Up

This chakra is all about seeing beyond your eyesight, seeing from your third eye, from your intuition. When your energy is balanced and flowing in this chakra, you are receiving an abundance of ideas and solutions. However, when you begin to worry, overanalyze, and become skeptical of intuition, you can easily block the flow of this vital guidance. If you're feeling unmotivated and stagnant, overwhelmed with your life, or absent in your relationship with others, you need to consider getting this chakra up and running again. To check your sixth chakra, honestly answer these questions:

- Do you have any health conditions related to the eyes, nose, brain, or neurological system?

- Do you usually forget your dreams?

- Do you tend to be closed-minded?

- Do you typically only see one way to address an issue?

- Do you deny or ignore the truth of a situation?

- Do you shut off or ignore inner guidance?

- Do you behave in a way that is against your own ethics and morality?

- Do you expect negative results from most situations?

- Do you have a hard time concentrating or focusing on tasks at hand?

- Do you often forget things you need to do?

- Do you overreact to situations rather than rationally try to deal with them?

If you answered yes to two or more of these questions, chances are your sixth chakra could use a tune-up.

How to Clear Sixth Chakra Blockages

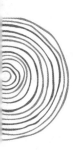

Clearing your sixth chakra opens the line of communication to your Higher Self. When you set the intention and make a commitment to listen inside, you honor the guidance you receive with suitable actions.

Since this chakra is highly visual, surround yourself with beauty and things that give you a feeling of inner harmony. A vase of flowers can do wonders. Also, take a little time each day to give your eyes a visual treat, either with captivating images of light and color or ones that are simply beautiful. Explore your neighborhood. Approach life with a sense of childlike wonder.

Before you go to sleep at night, set the intention to remember your dreams. When you can, jot down your dreams. You may want to keep a dream journal. Make note of any emotions or physical sensations you experienced during the dream. Look for recurring patterns. As you examine each element of your dream, see if you can figure out what your subconscious is trying to tell you.

Healing herbs and oils to enhance this chakra include sandalwood, star anise, mugwort, and saffron. Healing scents to take in are gardenia, lavender, and rosemary. You can also consume a small handful of sunflower seeds or a little wheat germ oil to boost this area. An amethyst crystal, bearing the sixth chakra color of lilac, can also improve energy and flow. When working with this delicate area of the body, you might want to try a crystal like kyanite for protection against individuals who may try to attack you psychically.

One of the most effective ways to strengthen this chakra is to honor your need for solitude. Being highly intuitive can often make you overly empathic, meaning you pick up way too much energy from others around you. You may need to avoid people and places that drain you. Spend more time by yourself. Turn off electronics, light candles and incense, meditate, read a book, just *be*. Solitude is the perfect way to replenish and recharge.

Another way you can develop and heal your sixth chakra is through visualization. Get in the practice of creating images on your internal mind screen and visualizing the results you desire in order to sharpen your skills. When approaching any problem, task, or goal, visualize a positive outcome. Strengthening your visualization skills will also strengthen your ability to see beyond this dimension.

Sixth Chakra Exercise: Sharpening Your Third Eye

This exercise is designed to strengthen your ability to "see" with the third eye. You can do this anytime you have a quiet moment, maybe at the end of your meditation practice. Sit comfortably with your eyes closed. You can use this exercise to look at a situation or problem from varying perspectives in order to arrive at a better picture of the truth. Afterward, you may want to write down all that you see and sense on each level. The example I use in this exercise is learning to look at a potential mate with clear inner sight.

Imagine you are climbing a pyramid. When you stand on the lowest step and look out, you are seeing from the first chakra, your base chakra for survival. What do you see when you look at this person you're interested in? What do you feel? Is he or she someone with whom you feel safe, protected, taken care of?

Climb to the next step and look out from the point of view of the second chakra, your sacral chakra that is the center of movement. What do you see this time? What do you feel? Are you turned on by this person? Are you moving in sync with each other? Or are you looking to this person to make you feel more complete?

As you ascend each step, you are sensing from the broader perspective of each higher chakra. As you reach the next step, you are looking out from the point of view of the third chakra, your power chakra. What do you see now? Does your potential mate acknowledge who you are and let you stand in your own power without trying to tear you down? Or does he or she need you to shore up his or her own weak self-esteem?

Climb to the next step and look out from the point of view of the fourth chakra, your heart chakra, for balance. What can you see here? Are you able to exchange warm and tender feelings with this person?

Now you are at the next step, looking out from the point of view of the fifth chakra, your throat chakra, for how you express what you see and feel from this view. This is a vital perspective for a successful relationship: Are you comfortable revealing your conflicting thoughts and deepest emotions to this person? Is there real communication between you?

When you climb to the step of the sixth chakra, you now have a much more panoramic view. Even though you may be looking at the same situation or scene, your perspective and the information you receive will be very different. Write down this new vision and compare it to the different levels. Notice how you're seeing much more on each higher level. Do you see any red flags warning you about this person? Is there any feeling in your gut that this person is not good for you?

When you reach the pinnacle of the pyramid, the seventh chakra, you are now looking through the panoramic eyes of mastery. Is this potential relationship for your highest good? Will it bring you higher in love and consciousness or drag you deeper down? Is this person a higher or lower vibration than your own?

Do this exercise again in a few days and notice if your perceptions of this person (or whatever the situation is that is the subject of this exercise) have changed.

Next, we're heading to the higher spiritual chakras, where you get directly connected to Source.

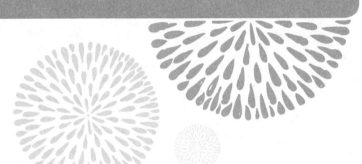

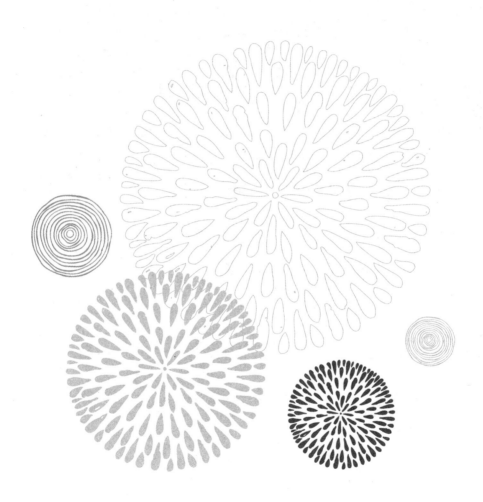

THE SEVENTH CHAKRA, THE SOUL STAR, AND BEYOND

Now we're ready to go to the "crown of creation"—the high spiritual chakras that are your direct connection to Source.

The Seventh Chakra—Knowing

The seventh chakra is called the crown chakra because it is located at the top of your head. In Sanskrit, the seventh chakra is called *sahasrara*, which means "thousandfold," as in the thousand-petal lotus that symbolizes a fully awakened seventh chakra. As a high vibrational energy center, the seventh chakra is a focal point during your quest for enlightenment. The more your crown chakra opens, the more you evolve as a conscious being. When this chakra is open and in balance, resonating in harmony with the other chakras, you can step across the portal into "cosmic consciousness," becoming one with the entire universe.

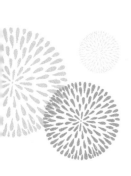

The crown chakra is important at both the beginning and end of life: it's the soft spot on a baby's skull (the opening where the soul enters the body) and the spot where the soul leaves the body at the moment of death. It connects to all aspects of mind—thought, intelligence, information, and consciousness—as well as to the larger Mind (divine intelligence) and the process of inner knowing.

The element of this chakra is thought—one of the ways in which the unified field of consciousness surrounds and flows through you. The information from your crown chakra goes beyond the data you receive from your standard five senses.

In the seventh chakra, the governing principle is order, the way you create internal patterning (the beliefs that influence what and how you perceive). In the seventh chakra, you shift away from your personal identity. Instead of asking, "Who am I?" the question becomes "What does it all mean?" In this chakra is the seat of the ultimate state of consciousness where you experience total unity with the universe and all others. Here you discover that the answers to all your questions lie within.

The crown chakra is the summit of the physical body's chakra system and the pinnacle of spirituality in the body. This chakra functions like a matchmaker—helping you to unite intimately with Source and experience the bliss and peace that passes all understanding. The energy that started off quietly coiled at the base of your spine can now climb to the top of your head. When this energy reaches the seventh chakra, you turn the switch for unity consciousness to "on." The higher up the ladder of consciousness you climb, the more you see and understand.

The Seventh Chakra's Biggest Obstacle

Problems commonly develop in the crown chakra around early adulthood and as you mature and broaden your wisdom. What is the obstacle that keeps you from receiving the ultimate wisdom of the universe? It's attachment. It's okay to have some healthy attachments to loved ones or positive goals. But when you want to relinquish your responsibilities, give in to your ego, control others, or force things to go your way without keeping an open mind, the energy channels in this chakra will slam shut.

To open these channels again, you need to release your hold on old and outmoded belief systems. This includes whatever happened to you when you were growing up, as well as your religious, political, and social opinions that no longer serve you. Your convictions are the filter through which you understand everything you experience, so if you want to change your life, you first have to reprogram beliefs that are harmful to you. If your interpretation of the world is based on a principle that was formed when you were traumatized as a child, you may be operating from a place of mistrust and fear. Examine your beliefs and see which ones are getting in the way of truly accepting and loving yourself.

The Health of Your Seventh Chakra

The seventh chakra is the key that unlocks the secrets of higher consciousness, taking you beyond thoughts and perceptions and into a highly tuned awareness. When your crown is open, you have faith in the transcendent realms and you have a sense of purpose in life. Here in the higher realms, you can understand the perfect pattern for your relationship to all beings, the universe, and Source. With an open crown chakra, you don't judge or criticize others but rather embody love, compassion, and awareness.

If the crown chakra is closed, you won't even understand what a spiritual experience is. If your crown chakra is deficient in energy, there may be an excess of energy in the lower chakras, creating a breeding ground for greed, materialism, and the desire to control others. Some classic life situations that can interfere with your seventh chakra include hanging around skeptics, needing to always be right, obsessing about material things, using recreational drugs, or abusing prescription drugs.

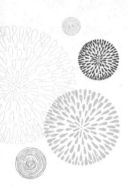

The crown chakra connects to both the pineal and pituitary glands deep in the brain and is associated with the hypothalamus, the central nervous system, and the right eye. Also, it is somewhat linked to your immune system as it relates to the psyche. The diseases or disorders that can come from an unbalanced seventh chakra are feeling alone and disconnected from others, anxiety, depression, insomnia, bipolar disorder, amnesia, headaches, strokes, brain tumors, epilepsy, multiple sclerosis, Parkinson's, attention deficit disorder and hyperactivity, amyotrophic lateral sclerosis (ALS), mental illness, and dementia or Alzheimer's disease.

Archetypes

The dysfunctional archetype for the crown chakra, when it is closed or unbalanced, is the egotist, who can be a success in the world but is too arrogant to allow the unfolding of her spirituality. Egotists are full of pride and feel they are so important that there couldn't possibly be any higher power than they. The egotist barrels through any problems using willpower and sheer force. In psychological terms, egotists are called narcissists—interested only in their own achievements, dramas, and ego. Egotists, unlike the first chakra victims, believe that they alone are responsible for everything they have accomplished.

The sage is the positive archetype of the crown chakra. The sage is a spiritual master at a high level of attainment—the embodiment of awareness, compassion, and unconditional love. There have always been teachers and healers who, rather than seeking power from outside of themselves, have channeled Source and known that their power comes from that higher place.

Attachment is the main obstacle standing between being who you are now and becoming the sage. This is tricky, since there are healthy attachments to loved ones, spiritual guides, and the goal of liberation—these are known as golden chains. But releasing the sticky parts of attachment doesn't mean you relinquish responsibility; rather, you no longer direct your energy to what is outside of you, such as a need to control others, and you release your attachment to the fruits of your efforts.

Spiritual Aspects

A lot of energy gets processed in the crown chakra, and that energy can stagnate if it gets stuck in your head. Since this chakra's sense organ is the central nervous system, when energy flows smoothly, the nervous system stays calm, your ability to think clearly improves, and you are happy to receive inspiration and guidance from above.

The seed sound for the crown chakra is *Visarga*, which is actually a particular type of breathing sound that, when used before meditation, unifies the smaller energy centers associated with the crown. For example, some Brahmins in the Hindu tradition have a tuft of hair at the back of the head at the location of the *Bindu visarga*, which is the source of *amrit*, the sweet nectar that drips down from the palate onto the tongue and spreads bliss throughout the body.

A fully opened crown chakra unites kundalini energy with the energy of Source; after a while, kundalini descends once more to the base chakra, leaving you in an expanded state of consciousness. You are now able to enter higher planes, including:

- The plane where *Om* is continuously heard

- The plane of enlightenment

- The plane where you can master the subtle energy of prana

- The plane of balance in body, mind, and spirit

- The plane of acknowledging Source and releasing judgmental mind and dualistic thinking

Uranus is the planet associated with the crown chakra. In astrology, Uranus rules the stars, freedom, and originality. Native American traditions say that we came from the stars, that Star Teachers formed their culture and spiritual beliefs, and that one day the Star Nations will return.[1]

Know When to Give Your Seventh Chakra a Tune-Up

The crown processes a lot of energy, and if that energy gets stuck in your head, it can stagnate. You feel overwhelmed. You become closed-minded when it comes to new challenges and experiences. Your opinion is the only one that matters to you. You are caught up in your own pride and self-importance. You'll feel you don't need anyone to help you; you'll think you can do it all on your own.

The sense organ for this chakra is the central nervous system. When your energy is flowing smoothly, the nervous system stays calm, you think clearly, and you welcome spiritual guidance and inspiration from above.

To fully awaken your crown chakra, your body, mind, and spirit must be in balance, with the energy flowing smoothly between the pineal gland and the right and left cerebral hemispheres. To check your crown chakra, honestly answer these questions:

- Do you distrust or not believe in your higher power?

- Do you feel like you've been abandoned?

- Do you tend to think that your beliefs are the only right ones?

- Do you feel unsupported by the universe?

- Do you feel alone and isolated?

- Do you feel as though your mind is foggy?

- Do you regularly feel overtired and like you are not getting enough sleep?

If you answered yes to three or more of these questions, chances are your seventh chakra could use a tune-up.

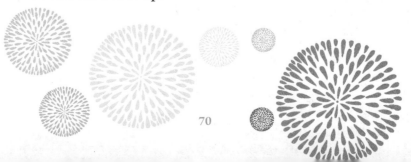

How to Clear Seventh Chakra Blockages

The main quality to cultivate in the seventh chakra is being mindful—simply paying attention to each moment without getting attached to any particular moment or outcome. The best way to open your crown chakra is through the regular practice of meditation, prayer, or ceremony that will strengthen your connection to the universal field of consciousness. These practices energize and calm your mind so you can enter higher states of consciousness.

Meditation may be the perfect practice for opening the crown chakra, but the real key is surrender. Your connection to Source can be blocked at any given time by anxiety, fear, and anger. When you find a way that works for you to release these difficult emotions, your crown chakra will open and you will live fully and be able to lead your life for the good of humankind. Honor the connection you already have with Source and greater levels of connection will open up.

The crown chakra can be seen as either white or gold. Quartz crystals are perfect for this chakra, as they contain the full range of light frequencies, illuminating the crown chakra and higher. Other stones for this chakra are amethyst and diamonds. You can use incense or essential oils like frankincense or myrrh to help open your crown chakra. And to best support this chakra, keep plenty of blueberries, eggs, and fish in your diet.

The Eighth Chakra—Higher Perception

You may be surprised to learn that the chakras don't end at number seven. The basic seven chakras—the ones that run from the base of your spine up to the top of your head—are all about your development here on earth. But there are a number of higher chakras that help you merge with your Higher Self and the entire universe. We are born with them, but these higher chakras must be unlocked by your spiritual progress along the path.

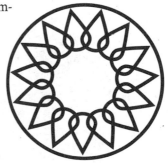

The eighth chakra, called the soul star, sits around two feet above the crown chakra. It acts as the center of the whole chakra system—protecting your physical, emotional, and spiritual bodies—and as the root of the divine energy that saturates your chakra system. Between the crown chakra and the eighth chakra is the Stellar Gateway, where divine light and energy come down into your seventh chakra so they can flow throughout your body. Here you can fully let go so the light of Spirit fills you, allowing you to transcend to higher realms. Someone who is vibrating at the level of the eighth chakra is what Buddhists call a *bodhisattva*—someone who is totally selfless and full of compassion. Bodhisattvas put aside their final merger with Source and agree to keep coming back to embodiment on earth until all sentient beings are liberated.

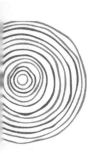

The eighth chakra looks like an orb, filled with light, and may have a white or slightly orange glow. The main color associated with this chakra, however, is ultraviolet light that you can't see with your physical eyes. Instead, visualize a deep violet light that has spiral bands of green. At times, I see a ray of white light when I'm looking at this chakra in someone. This is the clear light that aids in healing and spiritual cleansing and gives a powerful boost to emotional balancing, stability, and deep inner peace.

The eighth energy center is the first *transpersonal* chakra, which is associated with ascension, higher spiritual perceptions, and wisdom. Because you have moved beyond your limited self in accessing this chakra, you can sense your connection to a vast community of higher beings.

The symbol of the eighth chakra is the divine seed, or the blue pearl, a tiny blue light that switches on when the crown chakra is activated. In ancient Indian tradition, it is said that the blue pearl is the primary seed (or key) of life itself.

The Eighth Chakra's Biggest Obstacle

When this chakra is not yet activated, you feel separate from the rest of the world and from your soul purpose. The eighth chakra also holds your karmic residue—those life lessons that are stored in patterns of energy that you carry with you from previous experiences. Basically, this is the last energy center to

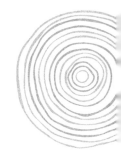

hold anything human. As you expand your consciousness and head out into the universe, it's time to annihilate any leftover negative behavior or thought patterns that keep you from moving forward on your quest for wisdom and guidance. It's only when you knock out negativity that you clear away your old patterns and open up your receptivity to the spiritual gifts and abilities you are meant to have.

The Health of Your Eighth Chakra

With each step you take farther into this realm, the closer you get to understanding your true destiny. Often while working with this eighth energy center, you connect with your spirit guides, including the mighty angels of the higher realms who will help in the activation of your ethereal or light body. Your Higher Self has always known your soul's purpose. Once you are in touch with your Higher Self, you can begin to recognize your soul's purpose. When you activate the eighth chakra, it downloads higher qualities that you want to develop—perhaps humility, courage, or patience—into your body and psyche so you can manifest those qualities now.

Know When to Give Your Eighth Chakra a Tune-Up

If you're stuck in your old ways, are closed-minded about changing anything, and see only the negative side of things, your eighth chakra is definitely due for some tuning up! Maybe you're an emotional wreck, trying to keep your feet on the ground as you search for some tranquility and peace of mind. You have the feeling that there's so much more to life, but you can't figure out your place and purpose in it. You're feeling alone and disconnected. Time for a tune-up!

How to Clear Eighth Chakra Blockages

Since you are at the Stellar Gateway getting ready to fly up to a transformational new realm of spiritual wisdom, your meditation practice is *mandatory* at this level. It's the only way to put your energy in balance and allow your mind, body, and soul to open wide and accept this ultimate level of your super power. Before your meditation, try chanting the mantra *Ma-ah-zod* for a minute or two. This will help clear out any karmic residue you're holding onto. Remember, mantras are the perfect tools to unlock the energy needed for healing.

When working with this soul star chakra, include some rare stones that are high vibrational crystals. Use clear quartz crystals or white selenite crystals, which are often used in healing wands, to activate this chakra. For more advanced energy healing, use tanzanite, amethyst crystals, and sugilite (a rare pink-to-purple stone). These help the white light from the etheric plane of Spirit to flow down throughout the entire body.

This soul chakra is a highly sensitive area. So if you're working with the eighth chakra of another person, remember to protect yourself from psychic attack. I recommend taking a clearing bath when you're done. (You'll find instructions for how to do this in chapter 13.) If for some reason you can't take a clearing bath right away, then you'll want to wash your hands and let the water flow over your wrists and fingers. This will help clear away any negative energies you may have picked up and will also break your contact with the other person.

Eighth Chakra Exercise: Soul Star Meditation

Find a quiet place where you can sit comfortably to do this meditation. Now close your eyes. Take a deep breath in through your nose and exhale. Take a few more deep breaths and release any tension or stress with each exhalation.

With the next couple of deep breaths, release any fear from your body. If you have any fear about anything, the eighth chakra will remain closed. Keep breathing. As you inhale, breathe in tranquility and calmness. As you exhale, breathe out any and all worries and concerns. To keep yourself protected from these worries and negative energy, imagine that you are covered in an egg-shaped golden light. This will give you another layer of strong protection against negativity and fear.

Now focus on the images that appear on your mind's screen and repeat the following mantra: *Aham prema* (pronounced *ah-HUM PRAY-ma*). This Sanskrit mantra means "I am divine love." When you repeat this mantra, it affirms your own love energy and activates the transformation and awakening of higher love within you.

Gently focus your attention on your first chakra, the root center. Visualize it as a field of red. Now slowly move up to your second chakra and picture it as a field of orange. Keep gently rising up to your solar plexus chakra and imagine it as a golden-yellow blaze. As you move up the chakras with your intentionality, you'll notice these colors will intensify in brightness and clarity.

Rise up further into the life-giving green glow of the heart chakra. Pause for a moment to acknowledge your thymus—the seat of your development that sits between the heart and throat chakras. Now rise again into the blue shimmer of the throat chakra, the shining purple ray of your third eye, and finally the white or gold light of your crown. Feel these chakras expand and open in both the front and the back of your body.

After you feel your entire chakra system opening and widening, visualize your energy funneling into a glimmering silver cord that comes up from your crown and disappears into the higher dimensions above.

Gently allow your awareness to rise up this cord to about two feet above your head, where your eighth chakra is located. Imagine opening a door into a beautiful room infused with white light. Bathe in its splendor. There is no one way the room should look; this inner sanctum will be unique to you.

Here, as you bathe in the light of the soul star chakra, you meet your Higher Self. Yes, you really are that magnificent! What are the questions

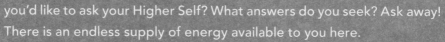

you'd like to ask your Higher Self? What answers do you seek? Ask away! There is an endless supply of energy available to you here.

Now gently bring the energy *down*, all the way from above your head into the crown chakra, letting it flow downward through all your chakras. Take this energy all the way down through each energy center—third eye, throat chakra, heart chakra, solar plexus, sacral chakra, and root chakra. Take it all the way to the bottom of your feet. Now anchor the energy in the earth below you.

Sit quietly as you feel your connection to the energy of the earth. Gently open your eyes.

Beyond the Eighth Chakra

The ninth chakra: Located about four feet above your head, the ninth chakra brings the energy of the Christ light into your inner and outer worlds. All your body's cells fill with joy and sparkling light, and the chakra looks like a spinning rainbow when it's fully open. This chakra is the home of your karmic blueprint, which contains all the skills you have developed over lifetimes. The three principal life blueprints are the creator, the teacher, and the healer. You may fit into more than one category, but the main one determines your destiny.

The tenth chakra: Here in the tenth chakra, you can begin to use everything you have learned in your previous lives. It doesn't matter if you were male or female in those past lives; in the tenth chakra you merge both genders, joining together the sun and moon principles. But if you still have fear in your energy field, it can keep the chakra from opening and functioning optimally. Since the tenth chakra is located at least eight to ten feet above your head, you have to focus on your intent to send healing energy to the chakra by way of the heart chakra. This chakra has multiple layers that may need healing. If the tenth is not cleared of blocked energy, all the other spiritual chakras will feel the effects. To heal the tenth chakra, it is necessary to dissolve your fears and release any energy blockages by holding an intense blue light in your mind while directing your attention to whatever needs to be cleared.

The eleventh chakra: Reaching the eleventh chakra indicates a very advanced level in your spiritual journey. You merged with the Mother aspect of the soul when the eighth to tenth chakras opened. As the eleventh and twelfth chakras open, you connect and unite with the Father aspect. You now exist on various planes of existence all at the same time. Your work is to go beyond the confusion of going into new dimensions in order to become more conscious on all planes. It commonly takes years before the spiritual chakras open up fully, with the eleventh and twelfth chakras taking the longest.

The twelfth chakra: At this level, you merge with the cosmos. If your third eye is open, you will enjoy the radiance of this chakra, which is located about twenty feet above your crown. It's like a vibrating sun of swirling colors— the source of your strength and power and your ability to manifest change in physical and nonphysical reality. In this chakra you have to face your fear of leaving the earth. Relax. It may take at least a lifetime!

And beyond: If only the twelfth chakra were the top of the whole energy system! But there are still more chakras to go. Just as chakras eight through twelve go into the fourth dimension, chakras thirteen through twenty-two are the energy centers for the fifth dimension, in which you offer yourself in service to humanity and all sentient beings. Then chakras twenty-three through twenty-nine are sixth-dimensional chakras, and it keeps going into the seventh dimension!

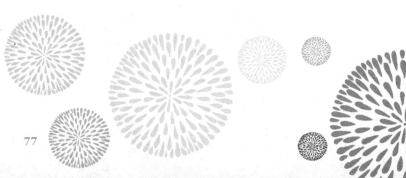

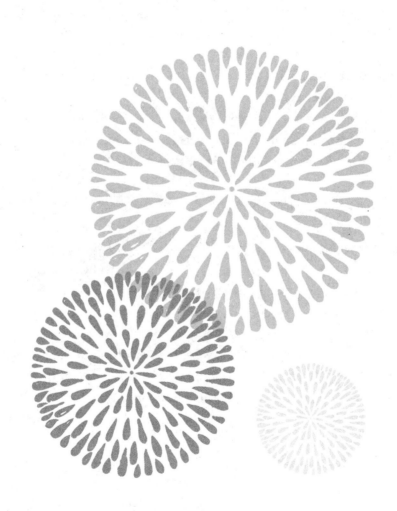

THE TRANSFORMATIVE
POWER OF INITIATION

There is a process that allows you to expand your healing consciousness and eventually merge back into Source—a long progression that takes place over many lifetimes. It's called initiation. Initiation encompasses all the step-ups in consciousness on the path to mastery. The higher your consciousness, the better you will be at healing with energy. Initiation brings more openness and balance, more consciousness, and more flowing energy, so you are more compassionate and more effective as a healer.

Your True Origin

Right now you are living your human life—the short encapsulated span of time that you are here in your earth suit. But let's start at the very beginning of your existence.

As many cultures and great thinkers teach, you actually began as a soul in a realm beyond this physical universe. Then one day, while you were floating around on another dimension, you decided you wanted to achieve a certain goal. Maybe the last time you were on earth, you betrayed someone and now you're going to work on being more loyal. Or maybe in another realm you were a coward and you want a chance to develop your courage and be more fearless. So you decide to incarnate and live here on earth again and try to learn your lessons a little better than last time.

Pop! Out you come into the world and, darn, you don't remember a thing about the lessons you came here to learn.

Even though you can't recall your true origin, you still have a yearning inside to do good unto others and to keep raising your vibration and consciousness. Then the reality of life kicks in and you're learning plenty of lessons and facing a whole series of new experiences, none of which are easy. Of course, you're always given a choice between the high road and the low road. You can be truthful or lie. You can admit your mistakes or blame others. You can be generous with your time and skills, or you can live as if it's all about you, all the time. When you make the right ethical decisions often enough, you are ready to initiate into higher levels of consciousness.

You may think of initiation as a rite of passage, a ceremony like baptism or a bar mitzvah that formally acknowledges your acceptance into a religious tradition. Or you might envision individuals wearing white robes, bringing flowers and incense to their spiritual preceptor as they become initiates into a particular sect or practice. Initiations into the "secret teachings" of the Great Mysteries go back to Atlantis, Egypt, Persia, India, Greece, and China as well as Europe and America. However, real initiation is not something that happens outside of yourself; it happens inside you.

Your initiation into the higher levels of consciousness is a shift in your perception, a new way of looking at "what is" in your life. The word *initiation* stems from the Latin, meaning "entrance" or "beginning." Quite literally, it means "going within." And that's the true nature of initiation into levels of higher wisdom—it allows you to go into your inner self, gaining entrance into a new level of awareness and beginning the next phase in your journey.

My Initiation into the Higher Levels of Consciousness

My experience with initiations began with my studies with various Christian healers. Initially, I spent several years in residence with an esoteric group of Christians who devoted themselves to emulating the message of the Christ in the New Testament: go out and heal. When I studied and practiced with these mystical Christians, I was amazed by how gifted they were. They often were purely selfless and strongly connected to Source, showing no signs of ego whatsoever. I noticed how quiet, discreet, and humble they appeared to be; when I would question them about their beliefs or the right way to live, they would guide me to discover the answer on my own. "Use your discernment," they would often say.

Some years later, when I was writing my thesis while working toward an advanced degree at a chakra-based healing school, I chose to follow and interview ten Christian ministers who conducted healing ceremonies. Like the esoteric Christians, some of these ministers were quite gifted at bringing in the Light.

Both groups—the esoteric Christians as well as the healing ministers—had an amazing ability to tap into divine energy, a sort of healing light that I could feel when I was around them. However, I also noticed that while they could attract and conduct that energy, they were not practiced at transmitting or aiming that energy at their intended subject. Instead, it often came into the room at random. Nor had these individuals had training in protecting themselves from negative forces. Finally, many of them seemed quite depleted by their work.

Despite these limitations, these Christians—both clergy and laypeople—had the strongest ability to attract divine energy I had seen in my worldwide study of energy healing. At that time, I was teaching at a well-established energy healing school in the United States. The techniques we taught at the school were valid, but I sensed that the connection to Source that was needed to fuel the techniques had been lost. Energy healers have to go beyond mere technique and implement a higher power into their healing work for the healing to be effective. Over time, I learned how to combine the two—the ability to attract, conduct, and transmit the light as well as to simultaneously utilize the healing school techniques, which included staying grounded and safe from dark energies.

The first initiation I ever witnessed happened while I was following one of the Christian ministers. I was sitting in the back of a church as the minister worked with a woman up front. All of a sudden, I felt a huge blast of energy that simultaneously knocked me to my knees and made me feel like I was going to fly through the air. I turned to a woman sitting near me and whispered, "What just happened up front?" She said, "Oh, we call that an initiation."

I spoke to one of my esoteric Christian teachers about this incident, and she told me that I'd be facilitating these types of experiences myself—that it was to be my gift. At the time I hadn't been working in the field very long, and I found her comment unbelievable. I didn't think I had the talent, yet deep inside I knew how much I wanted to do this very thing. I kept working on myself to prepare for this next step. I studied, I prayed, I fasted, I meditated, and I was of service wherever and whenever the need arose. Finally, one day, I could not only sense the initiatory energies, but I could also bring them in. Over many years and thousands and thousands of initiations, I not only mastered attracting that divine energy but also learned how to conduct and transmit it to a specific individual and how to ensure that the person doesn't lose it later. That in itself is a very tricky step. More recently, I learned how to transmit this divine energy to a group and how to transmit it via video. Who knows what the next refinement will be!

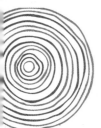

The Doorway to Your Higher Life

When this energy is transmitted to you, what does it mean for you personally? To answer that question, let me first tell you all about the initiatory levels.

Everyone starts out on the first level—the survival level. You remember being there: all you cared about was surviving, worrying about your job, your partner, your appearance. Initiation opens the doorway for new energies to unfold and assimilate into your awareness and your life, allowing you to progress to higher levels of being, where you have an expanded awareness. It does take time, sometimes years, to move up from one level to the next. For example, say you've been taking care of your aged mother for many years, but your service has felt like obligation and you've not been happy doing it. With your newly expanded awareness, you can now see that your mother is really an aspect of yourself and that caring for her is also taking care of yourself. Now you can hang out like two souls instead of butting heads on a personality level. You have more peace and equanimity, and you do your caregiver job with more grace. As you go up in levels of awareness, your relationships with everyone around you will change because your perspective now includes more compassion and a greater understanding of the issues facing the other person.

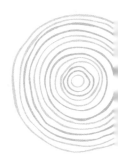

Energy healing, in order to be effective, needs to be done from the highest level possible. Jesus, the Christ, the most effective healer in modern history, is also the highest initiate we know of. Wouldn't you love to be able to heal an entire crowd like he could? I know I would. I've never seen anyone else with the ability to do that.

Initiation really comes down to expanding your energy field with a constant inflow of wisdom and knowledge. Think of your field as a giant bubble and, as you're sitting in it, it gets larger and larger. As you expand your desire to learn more ways to help others, your soul will expand and you'll start picking up messages and vibrations from your divine Higher Self. That's why the healing circles we'll talk about at the end of this book are a major way to foster more healing energy for you and for the world; they are like ever-expanding bubbles of consciousness and good will.

The First Seven Levels of Initiation

There are different ways of describing the process of initiation that leads to realization of self and God on the journey to enlightenment. It's a gradual spiritual evolution, not a series of physical events, although some initiations feel very physical indeed!

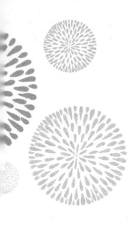

There are 352 levels of initiation that one takes when following the journey back to Source.[1] However, I will discuss only the first seven, since they make up the first round of the ascension process and what most people are likely to encounter in a single lifetime.

Over time, as you take initiation into higher levels of consciousness, you have to become more responsible for how you live your life. You are expected to be impeccable in truth and integrity, and responsible for the gifts you receive as you learn to maintain the higher frequencies brought through the initiatory process. For someone interested in energy healing, initiations hold the gift of healing.

The First Initiation: Physical Self—Birth

The first initiation represents the physical self and may happen at any powerful moment in your life—while being intimate with a partner, while giving birth, or while tending to someone who is dying. This first initiation may also occur while you are having a moment in nature, perhaps while running or skiing or sitting, watching the waves roll in, when for a moment you feel everyone and everything is connected.

After this initiation, you feel more connected to Source and have the desire to do good for others rather than always being solely focused on yourself. You may discover your personal path and start to seek out spiritual books, companions, and teachers. You begin to learn to control the hungers of the physical body, such as food, sex, and security. You may feel grateful not only for your life but also for all life in the natural world. Both this initiation and the second one described below can happen spontaneously at any time. Think back—chances are, you'll remember your own first or second initiation.

The Second Initiation: Emotional Self—Baptism

The second initiation represents the emotional self and opens you to divine love, stirring your desire to know your true self. It starts bringing your emotions and desires under more conscious control.

The biggest stumbling block for receiving this initiation is failing to love yourself—a common and very destructive problem. When you take control over your emotional body and take responsibility for yourself, you'll be open to this initiation. That's because you'll no longer feel like a victim or blame others for anything that goes wrong in your life.

I clearly remember my second initiation. I was in a yearlong program studying an advanced teaching program in meditation and had one month to go. One day in the meditation hall, we were sitting in silence, eyes closed, mentally repeating a strong mantra we had just received. Suddenly I started feeling heat radiating up from my hands, through my arms and neck, into my head. I was puzzled, knowing I was much too young to be having hot flashes.

Suddenly I "saw" in my mind that the seventy-five meditators in the room were connected. More than just connected, we were all *one*. It was an incredible moment. There was only one heart beating inside me at that moment, and it contained the hearts of all of us in that room. This glimpse into this unified field and the feelings it gave me were breathtaking.

The Third Initiation: The Soul Merge

For the sincere seeker, the time between the second and third initiations is often the hardest. This is because all the unbalanced aspects of the ego-bound personality begin to emerge here. However, at this point you are clearer about your own issues, and you are mostly free from being caught up in the illusion of the world. That's when you're ready for the third initiation, which is called the soul merge. You start to develop some mastery over your rational mind and thoughts, and you are far more aware of your ego-based issues. You also start releasing old blockages and distortions from the chakras.

During this third initiation, the soul star (the eighth chakra, see chapter 7) sends its light down through the top of your head and throughout the chakras, coming out the feet to anchor in the core of the earth. Your soul's light, energy, and consciousness merge with your physical body, bringing your soul to earth. This is truly being present in your body and is the beginning of living from a soul-based awareness. From here on in, the choices you make in your life will be based on the consciousness of your soul rather than on the desires of your lower chakras.

The Fourth Initiation: The Crucifixion

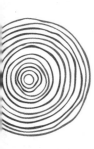

By the time you are ready for the fourth initiation, you are identifying with your soul instead of your ego. Your seventh chakra, at the crown, is open and getting purified. Initiation at this level can be an ecstatic experience. The "membrane" of the soul star gets absorbed into the twelfth chakra, way above your head. The soul star downloads everything it has understood from experiences in previous lifetimes. You may even be able to remember your past lives.

Now things are speeding up. At this stage, you want a deeper and fuller self-knowledge. The mighty I AM presence—Spirit—becomes your main guide. Renunciation begins on this level—in which you let go of clinging to all the ways you built your ego through power, wealth, status, appearance, and sex. Everything is stripped away. This is also the level where your higher mind unites the soul and Spirit. Here you dedicate your life to humanity rather than to the ideal of personal liberation. Those who become such channels of Spirit often sacrifice their lives to accomplish their missions, such as Jesus, Mahatma Gandhi, and Martin Luther King Jr.

The Fifth Initiation: Atma or Atmic (Higher Self)— Mastery

At the fifth level, the energy that comes from the light-filled heart of the soul star is downloaded into your heart. In turn, this activates the link between your heart and your thymus, and between your energy field and your physical body. This infusion of higher consciousness begins solar consciousness, which purifies the remnants of unworthiness from your heart. Here you get the first brief look at ascension, in which the earthbound personality, the soul, and the great I AM become unified on earth. You are now a "baby" Master.

The Sixth Initiation: Monad (God Self)—Decision

In the sixth initiation, you actually connect to ascension and enter into the fifth dimension. Here you have complete access to all that the unified field has to offer, and you begin to learn how to use the energies of light. Now you can more easily heal others on the physical level. At this point, you have a choice: you can leave the earth plane or stay in order to serve humanity. You will be more filled with Light, more bliss filled, and more deeply connected to Source and to the Ascended Masters. You will also be able to choose which path of higher evolution best suits you (based on the seven rays of the Ascended Master teachings: power, wisdom, love, peace, truth, abundance, and justice).

The Seventh Initiation: Logoic (Cosmic Self)—Resurrection

You are now completely liberated from earthbound functions and are further developing your ascension abilities. The seventh initiation is the highest one you can reach while on earth. Those who reach the seventh level are World Teachers. Energy implodes in their heart center; all the chakras turn into a column of scintillating light. Here you become totally committed to service and begin to have the ability to transcend physical laws. This is resurrection, so called because you have returned to Source as a child of God, a state of being filled with peace and tranquility. This also begins an association with extraplanetary existence.

After these seven levels have been achieved, everything that was experienced during the initiatory process on the physical plane is revisited during astral, solar, galactic, universal, and multiuniversal ascension. Each new step on the path of ascension is followed by another level of initiation. Each new level brings more power, love, and wisdom into your practice of energy healing.

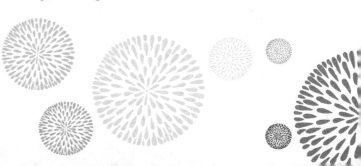

Near-Death Experiences

The first two levels of initiation are known as initiations of the threshold. They are like standing in a doorway and seeing a bright white light in the distance that is beckoning you forward. Sounds a little like a description of a near-death experience, doesn't it?

Actually, initiations can happen spontaneously during a near-death experience. A near-death experience happens when you are in the process of dying but death is aborted at the last second. You see a tractor trailer heading for your car; you go into cardiac arrest during a heart attack; you get caught in the undertow at the beach and start to drown; you are having surgery when you suddenly feel like you are looking down on yourself from the ceiling, watching the doctors as they try to restart your heart.

Surprisingly, during the near-death experience, you feel at peace, secure, warm, pain-free, and detached from your body. You may see a dark tunnel with a light at the end to which you keep moving closer. You may experience a review of your life as it flashes before you. Then you may hear a clear voice tell you it is not yet your time, that you have to go back, no matter how reluctant you are to leave the light or how broken your body that you now have to reinhabit may be. Or you may meet a Being of Light, an inner plane guide, or a deceased loved one who gives you that same message. Then, there you are, back in your body!

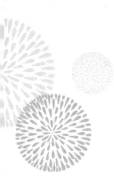

The fascinating thing about near-death experiences is the way in which they show that consciousness continues even when the heart stops beating or brain activity has flatlined. And even more interesting is the way in which having a near-death experience changes one's life. Those who "come back" from the dead have a renewed appreciation of life and a strong motivation to help others. They may now know their purpose in being here on earth, and they are willing to take on the responsibility of being a better person. In other words, they are experiencing the aftereffects of a spiritual initiation!

I have had three near-death experiences—two in which I almost drowned and one when I almost fell off a mountain.

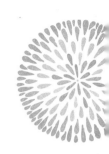

When I was barely twenty years old, I went on my first trip to Europe with my now husband, Eric, to visit his family in France and to climb mountains. Eric was a world-class mountaineer, certified as a Chamonix guide—a prestigious certification as a high mountain climbing guide. I was not. I'd only been mountain climbing for a year, and I was forever trying to keep up. California mountains are very gentle compared to the Alps. In the Alps, however, there is safety in numbers, and we would be climbing with two other teams, two people on each of the three ropes—five experienced climbers and me.

First we drove madly, in the French tradition, on a narrow road to a high village around 9,000 feet up—a village of old stone houses that seemed to date back centuries. There, we camped. We left at one o'clock the next morning so the glacier would still be firm when we crossed it. Glaciers in the Alps are far more serious than the ones in California, which could be crossed in an hour. Here they were gigantic, and if you were crossing one too late in the day, you risked falling into a crevasse. So we woke at midnight to leave the village.

Suddenly I had this strong premonition. I told Eric, "We can't go. Something horrible is going to happen today."

Eric said, "We'll just be very careful."

We started hiking straight up the mountain and arrived at the glacier around 2:00 a.m. It was still dark, and the glacier went straight up, so it was really scary. We put on crampons and got our ice axes out of our backpacks. We put on helmets with lights on them so we could see, and we roped up. If one of us fell into a crevasse, the other one on the rope would hope to stop their fall. And indeed, one of the team members promptly fell into a crevasse, and I got to see a rescue, which I realized I wasn't competent enough to handle for my own fellow climber. My heart was already in my throat, and at this point I just got more nervous. We got to the far side of the glacier just as the sun was coming up.

Suddenly two helicopters flew over, quite close to us. Half an hour later they came back. They had come to pick up the bodies of two dead climbers who had fallen on the rock cliffs ahead. This mountain was no joke, and we were headed to the top despite the fact that rescuers had just taken a couple of dead bodies off of it.

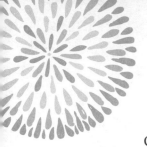

After the glacier, we were on friable rock, which is loose and unstable. In California, when I'd climbed in the High Sierra, rock faces tended to be pretty firm. This loose rock was another reason for me to be very alert. About two in afternoon, I was bone tired. By mistake, I dislodged something and a boulder above me—about the size of a Volkswagen Beetle—tumbled straight toward my head. Desperately praying that the rope would hold me, I instinctively threw myself off the face of the mountain to get away from the huge rock. As I pushed myself out over the abyss, I went into another state of consciousness, certain I was about to die!

The boulder came barreling past me and grazed my knee. Miraculously, I had landed on a platform. Eric was above me and couldn't see me. He felt the rope go slack and thought it had been cut by the bolder and I had fallen all the way, several thousand feet back down to the glacier, and was dead. Then he heard me screaming. The boulder had done more than graze my knee. There was a hole in my pants leg, and my leg muscle was destroyed. I couldn't use that leg. We weren't yet at the top of the mountain, and we had to get there in order to go down the other, more gentle side; there was no way to down-climb what we had just come up.

To top it off, a storm hit. In California, you can see the weather coming for several hours, but in the Alps, the mountains often hide the approaching storm until it bears down upon you. There was so much lightning that my ice ax "lit up," and I could hear a humming and buzzing in the air. Storms in the Alps are serious business! My five fellow climbers strung up ropes, and I had to get out of there by dragging myself endlessly, arm over arm, up the fixed ropes. My mistake had put the lives of the other five climbers at risk. We battled our way through the bad weather to the top and down the other side. Instead of being a fifteen-hour climb, it took us twenty-four hours.

I spent the rest of my summer in the hospital in France. It wasn't until some years later that I realized I had had a spiritual initiation back there on that mountain.

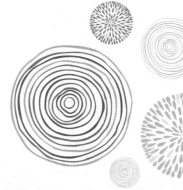

Beginning Your Initiatory Process

For the first two levels, you usually initiate on your own. Maybe you were walking on the beach and had one of those aha moments. Perhaps you had an epiphany about your life while attending a memorial for someone whose life was cut short, or maybe you felt inspired after an intimate moment with your soul mate. These are times when you feel so connected to everything, like the pieces of the puzzle are finally coming together. You start getting out of the survival level when you can handle your divorce without seeking revenge, when you accept the loss of your job without self-incrimination, or when you stop hoarding or bingeing. In other words, when you make the kind of decisions that enhance your awareness rather than hinder it with negative thoughts and behaviors, and when you couple it with any sort of service, that's when you're ready to initiate.

To reach the third level of initiation and above, however, you need a facilitator like me. You want to work with someone who's well trained and who comes from the heart rather than the ego to prepare you for your next step up the ladder of consciousness.

The Initiation of Jacques

Jacques attended one of my workshops. I noticed right away that he had a very strong meditative quality about him. He was a bit quiet, but you could feel a deeper power within him. I felt he was ready to initiate to the third level (which is not uncommon with my students, who are often seekers who have done much self-work); I could sense that readiness in his thymus, which is the seat of our spiritual development.

Jacques volunteered to come up to the front of the room to work with me. As he approached, I could sense a ball of light descending toward the top of his head. I synced my vibration to the level of the approaching energy, so I could *attract* it. My energy field enlarged so I could contain that energy within my own energy field. Around this same time, my heart chakra widened to absorb the energy. I pulled the energy in and, running it through my own energy field, I then *conducted* and *transmitted* it to Jacques. Using unbending intent, I brought the energy down his vertical power current (where his spine was located) and lodged it in his feet and then down into the earth. That way, he wouldn't be likely to lose the initiatory energy. Jacques said the experience gave him feelings of energy like bubbles of champagne running through him as he returned to his seat. (Every initiation is different, and each person experiences it differently.)

Later, I explained to Jacques and the others in the workshop that it is possible to lose an initiation. Every new initiate receives three tests, and if you fail all three, you can lose that new expansion and go back to the way you were before. The lost level of initiation is very hard, if not impossible, to regain later. I told them my own embarrassing story. I had taken an initiation while I was away from the healing school for the summer. Upon my return, I was bragging to my fellow teachers about my big initiation when the seer who led the school came into the room. He saw "ego" stamped all over me and banished me to the kitchen, far from the healing tables, to peel potatoes for a full year. Thanks to his swift action, he saved me from losing my initiation, and I'm here to help you do the same.

Your Advanced Gifts

As you no doubt have gleaned from the explanation of the seven levels, as a result of initiations, you become more open to the gifts we label paranormal—beyond what the average person knows, sees, thinks, or feels. These gifts are built into your cellular memory and into the collective unconscious. These amazing capabilities are part of being human. You probably already use some of these gifts without realizing it. You *intuit* who is calling before you answer the phone. You sense that your child is in trouble before the school calls you. Perhaps you refrain from renting or buying a particular house or apartment because you just *know* it feels wrong.

These gifts are beyond counting. Perhaps you have an innate gift of foretelling, knowing what's going to happen in the future, or you might have really strong intuitive abilities. Maybe you are clairvoyant and thus able to see on other planes. Perhaps you are meant to speak, teach, or heal at a high level. You may be aware of one or a few of the gifts you are meant to express. But that's one of the promises of working with energy—you have the power to open yourself up and allow your special gifts to flourish. You'll work first with the ones you already sense you have, as they will be your strongest gifts, but as we've seen, you have others waiting in the wings.

In part II, I am going to give you some of the best tools I know for expanding your consciousness, planting your feet firmly on the spiritual path, and enhancing your ability to heal yourself and, eventually, others.

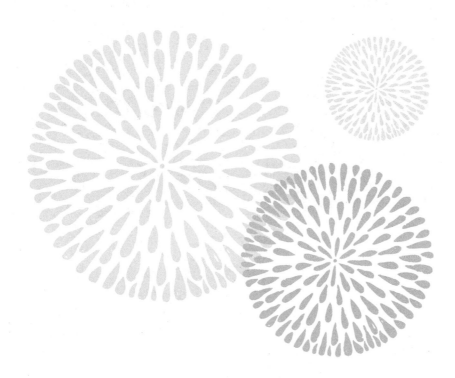

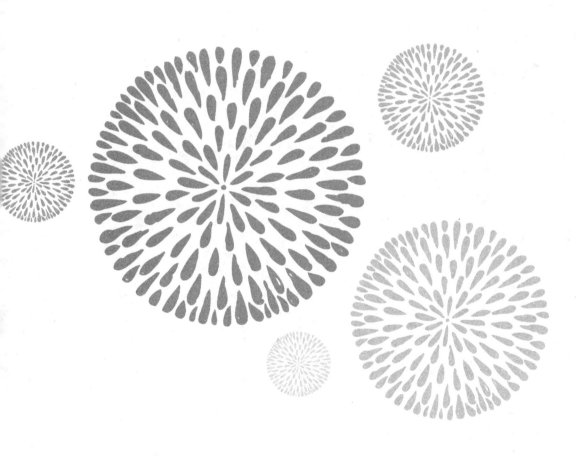

PART II

YOUR ENERGY
HEALING TOOLS

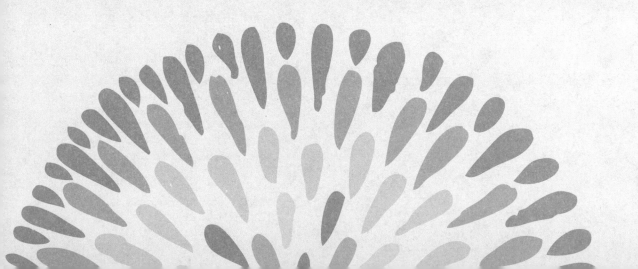

YOUR ULTIMATE ENERGY
TOOL: MEDITATION

Before you started reading this book, I bet you had no idea of the power you possess or the healing you can perform on yourself, and eventually perform on others. I've already taught you about the power of energy healing and how it works, where this power comes from, and how you can activate it in your life. We've covered the chakras—your seven energy centers in the body and the eighth chakra above your head (and some even beyond that)—and their importance for healing. Throughout the remainder of this book, I am going to share some uniquely powerful tools that I learned and mastered in my personal pursuit to become an energy healer. Each tool will help you strengthen and guide your inner power to all things healing and good.

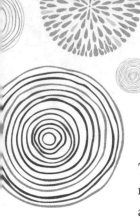

Meditation

The first energy healing tool I want to teach you about, and one that is your ultimate healing device, is meditation. You've most likely heard all about meditation and its benefits, but let me tell you even more.

The word *meditation* comes from the Latin root *meditatum*, which means "to ponder." It's a practice that focuses your attention inward, calms your mind, and has a wide range of powers to transform and heal you—emotionally, physically, and mentally. There is no downside to meditation. It has been practiced in the East for thousands and thousands of years and has of late solidly landed in the West.

Some forms of meditation have their roots in religious traditions, particularly Eastern ones: Buddhism, Hinduism, and Taoism. But you don't have to be involved in any religion to practice these meditation techniques; they all have the power to help heal you on many levels and help you grow in consciousness and compassion. You will really be amazed at how twenty minutes of meditation, once or twice a day, can power up your life.

You may have an image of meditation as someone sitting cross-legged on a cushion in full lotus position with incense wafting through the air. It can be so much simpler than that. With the right practice, you can just as easily sit in a cozy chair or your car (with your back straight), close your eyes (if you're not driving), and bask in a few minutes of being in the zone. That's it. You never even have to light a stick of sandalwood. Meditation is what you make of it and what's most comfortable for you.

The goal of meditation is to tune in to yourself, not shut off your mind or run away from troublesome thoughts. By closing your eyes and going inside, you will see yourself more clearly, and solutions to your problems will arise naturally. Meditation is excellent for de-stressing, relaxing, and helping bring you into a healthy state. Meditating can take you deeper spiritually, where you can connect to Source, as well as balance your chakras on every level.

Meditation's ability to help you tune in is why it is an important tool for energy healing: it focuses your attention on your consciousness, lets you get into the gap between your thoughts, and connects you to the universal energy field.

When anyone asks me the secret to my light-filled, healing life, my first response is always, "Meditation." As a spiritual teacher and energy healer, my number one recommendation to advance your pursuit of energy healing is a daily meditation practice. And I'm not just talking about sitting still for five or ten minutes each day or listening to soothing music or guided meditations. When you have learned to focus on a single object—and I use mantras for this purpose—you become more present with yourself, just as you are.

Meditation will take you deep into the inner silence and profound stillness of the universal energy field. This is exceedingly important because it allows you to connect not only with your Higher Self but also with the rest of the world. Imagine what the world would be like if we were all connected through meditation!

If you have a great deal of stored-up stress, as I did when I first started meditating, it may be a while before you can go this deep. But even when you first begin a meditation practice, you'll feel the healing benefits right away. Meditation immediately begins to raise your consciousness and helps you to release old energy from traumas or negative energy you've taken on in your life thus far.

As I mentioned earlier, when I was a competitive young lawyer in my twenties, busily climbing the grueling ladder of success at the cost of my health, I thought I was just fine. I justified my addictions as temporary or as a means to an end. But there was no end in sight. Each rung up the ladder led to another challenging step: making more money, getting even thinner, or winning the next big case. When I was diagnosed with cancer, I was forced to face myself—not an easy task. I was overwhelmed by fear about my health and about everything I had to do to get well.

This was an incredibly stressful time for me. So to keep from self-destructing, I started meditating: twenty minutes in the morning and then twenty minutes again later in the afternoon. It only took a couple of weeks before I noticed a big difference in my life. Every day, I used to walk out the front door of my house and get in my car to go to work. On one particular day after I started meditating, I walked out the same door as I always did and suddenly noticed these exquisite flowers growing in my front yard. I didn't know where they had come from until

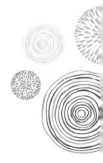

I realized I had planted these perennials myself the previous year. They'd been blooming for weeks, but I hadn't even seen them because I had been so preoccupied. Meditation allowed me to let in the world around me and taught me to be more open and less fearful. I have meditated every single day since.

Everyone has some problem to heal—a disease or health condition, anxiety and stress, difficulties with sleep, general unhappiness and lack of vitality, or old energetic blockages that keep them from functioning and feeling at their best. When you are ready to shift, to change in some fundamental way, turn to meditation as your number one tool.

With a continued meditation practice, all aspects of your life will become a lot easier. You'll be less reactive to external forces, more thoughtful, more present, happier, and healthier. Meditation is the best tool you can use to access your energy healing, and mantra meditation is one of the most effective methods.

Until you have a mantra, you can practice mindful breathing; it's an excellent exercise to prepare you for meditation.

Exercise: Mindful Breathing

Sit comfortably with a straight back, close your eyes, and put your attention on your breath. Feel your breath as it comes into your nostrils when you inhale and as it leaves your nostrils when you exhale. In other words, your awareness is "sitting" at the doorway of the nostrils and noting the breath as it goes in and out. Rather than try to follow the breath as it expands into your lungs, simply sit at the doorway and watch and feel the inhalation and exhalation.

What will it feel like? That depends on you. The breath might be hitting a particular part of the nostril. It may feel as light as a feather as it brushes past the nostrils, or it might seem to be throbbing. It might feel like intense pressure on your upper lip. There is no right or wrong way to breathe, and there is nothing to control. Just watch the breath and feel it.

Naturally, your mind will wander. You'll be bored. You'll get caught in thoughts or distracted by noises around you or sensations in your body. It's amazing how powerful an itch can be! Simply return your attention to your breath and its natural rhythm. If you find it difficult to keep your focus on the breath, try counting each breath till you get up to ten, then start again. Instead of trying to banish your thoughts, gently release them and keep on coming back to your breath.

Several minutes of mindful breathing will set you up for a good meditation, so let's go right into learning about the form of meditation I have found to be the most effective. The practice I teach is called LifeForce Meditation, which is a mantra-based type of meditation.

Mantra Meditation

A mantra is a sacred syllable or a word that you repeat to yourself internally so you can focus your mind. In other words, instead of paying attention to your breath, you will be paying attention to your mantra. Thank goodness, so much easier! The word *mantra* itself comes from Sanskrit and combines *man* (mind) and *tra* (liberate), so a mantra can *liberate your mind* with its vibrational energy.

A mantra in this sense is not the same as using an affirmation to keep you focused on a certain outcome, like *I am happy, healthy, and whole*; instead, it is more of a subtle driving wedge based on ancient Sanskrit seed syllables that will help you break through into higher levels of consciousness. Having a mantra will enable you to enter a very deep state of meditation. Coming from the ancient Vedic tradition, the sound of these mantras can transport you right into the unified energy field, more than concentration on the breath or visualizations can do.

The mantra you use and its pronunciation are very important, so you need to be given a mantra that is the right vibration that will connect you to Source.

Seed syllables plug you into your highest power—the Source of all wellness—and recharge you on every level. Once you receive your mantra, know that it is sacred and needs to be kept private and treated with respect. It should not be said aloud or shared with others. Until you are able to get your own mantra (check out the resource section for more information on obtaining your personal mantra on my website), you can use the generic seed syllable of *Om* as your mantra.

Calm Those Wild Thoughts

Here's a cool thing about meditation: it slows down those endless thoughts that continually bombard your mind. Our "monkey mind" is always chattering away—it's what the thinking mind does—and we can get caught in these loops of thoughts constantly playing and replaying in our mind.

In mantra-based meditation, you don't *stop* your thoughts. That's impossible. It's the mind's job to think. What meditation does is give you more space around your thoughts so you can see them more clearly after you've finished your meditation. Once you have this keener sense of awareness of your thoughts, you will automatically start to discard the ones that don't serve you. That goes for any bad or antiquated thoughts you might have about yourself too. A meditative practice sets you up to later see the workings of your mind—especially negative thought patterns—and effortlessly replace them.

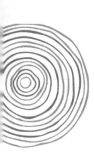

When you get to *know yourself* better as a result of meditation and can see and reflect clearly on your thoughts, you'll discover the benefits this practice can give you—a sense of calm, a feeling of abiding peace, and a sense of oneness with the rest of the world. With meditation, you can find yourself slipping into the space between your thoughts and resting in the universal energy field.

A regular meditation practice will beat any other relaxation technique to release your stress, improve your health, release your feelings of depression, give you an energetic face-lift, and all in all improve your quality of life. How super is that!

When Dark Thoughts Surface

If you are new to the practice of meditation, you may find that negative thoughts—the ones that you buried earlier in your life—surface during or after meditation. Don't worry; that's sometimes part of the process. If this happens, take a moment to observe your emotions quietly in a nonjudgmental way. It's normal for thoughts and feelings like this to arise, as the process of meditation clears old emotions and memories from your energy field, making you fresh and new. Send forgiveness to any individuals who may have harmed you, and certainly forgive yourself for your mistakes and any negative experiences you've had. This is part of the journey to self-mastery. If you can relax about your negative states and are unafraid to examine them closely, you'll be able to win your battle over guilt, shame, jealousy, anger, or any other tough emotion.

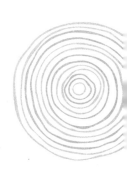

Here's what else I love about meditation: it connects you to that still, small voice of your inner knowing. You will be able to hear if you're heading in the wrong direction in your life. You'll have a clear sense if your relationship is worth saving. You'll know if there is an opportunity you need to explore further. Your inner voice will get louder as a result of meditation, and this voice will bolster your trust in yourself and your decisions. You will ultimately understand what you need to live your best life.

Your ability to connect to higher levels of thinking and higher planes of the universe will also develop in meditation. As you become more and more practiced and proficient, this information will make more sense to you. Your clearest perceptions usually happen after meditation, not during. You might be showering, having breakfast, or walking the dog when you are struck by powerful ideas and insights.

Here's the best part about meditation and why it's the ultimate energy-healing tool. As you already know, the higher up the spiritual ladder you climb, the more you come to realize the importance of helping others as well as yourself. Through a consistent meditation practice, you can actually help everyone on the planet. Whenever you hear, see, or read distressing news, you can do your part by meditating and sending out peaceful and healing vibrations as you meditate. By letting your higher consciousness ripple through the universal energy field in meditation, you are sending good, healing energy to everyone on the planet and ultimately healing the world. Now that's what I call energy healing!

In the next chapter, you'll learn how to meditate.

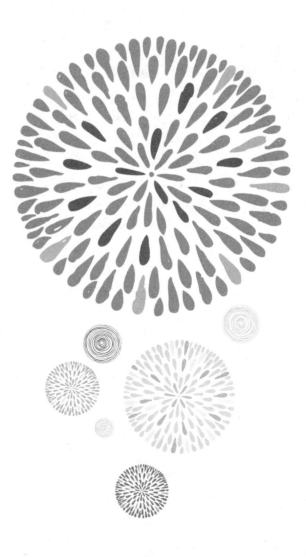

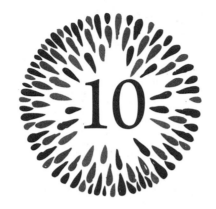

HOW TO USE MEDITATION
TO HEAL YOURSELF

You don't need to move into a secluded cave or to the top of a remote mountain to learn how to meditate. All you need to do is sit in a quiet place once or twice a day and follow a few basic recommendations. The following recommendations will help you get the most out of your practice. They will also give you the ideal way to go about establishing a meditation practice.

Meditate Every Day

It is only with consistent practice of meditation—twenty minutes once or twice a day, every day—that meditation works. It is an incremental practice that only works if done daily. Initially, the practice affects the "software" of your brain. Done regularly over five years, studies show that meditation can also affect the

"hardware" of the brain. A study by a neuroscientist at Harvard Medical School found that after participants meditated for twenty minutes twice a day even for just a couple of months, brain volume increased in four different regions of the brain connected with learning and memory, empathy, self-relevance, and emotional regulation as well as the part of the brain stem that produces neurotransmitters. Researchers also found that the part of the brain involved in the fight-or-flight response got smaller, reducing stress levels, anxiety, and fear.[1] Over time, you will find that meditation leads to a slower heart rate, improved sleep, and reduced blood pressure. Everyone can learn to meditate, and it becomes easier the longer you practice. It helps to schedule your meditation and do it around the same time every day.

When to Meditate

Meditate first thing in the morning! That means before exercise, before checking email and social media, before breakfast, and (gulp) even before your first cup of coffee. Early morning, right around sunrise, is the most powerful time of day to connect with your Higher Self. Ideally, you should plan to do your second meditation, when you have the time, right after work and before dinner. If you have an office, close the door and ask not to be disturbed. Or before starting your drive home, sit in your car and meditate. However, keep in mind that meditating too late in the day can adversely affect your sleep; you will want to meditate before dinner, not after.

You may not be able to add more hours to the day, but meditation will make it seem like you have because your ability to focus will likely increase, leading to greater productivity. As counterintuitive as it may seem, you're too busy *not* to sit down and "do nothing" once or twice a day for twenty minutes. You will soon find yourself looking forward to this downtime each day.

Get Your Body Ready

Sit in a chair or on a cushion or even in your parked car if it's the one place you can find solitude. Keep your back straight. Don't try to meditate while lying down or slumping on the couch. These positions signal to your body to go to sleep. You may want to use something to support your back, if you don't have a chair available, so you are not straining to stay erect. Close your eyes. There's less likelihood of getting distracted by something in your visual field, and it's easier to turn inward when you're not looking outward.

Eliminate or Ignore Distractions

Sounds from outside and your internal dialogue can all be distracting. Your body can also distract you with itching, minor pains, tingling, or strange sensations. Some distractions might even be the result of the meditation itself. You might see faces or images connected to old traumas; you might hear internal sounds, like crickets or bells or even beautiful melodies. This is all normal de-stressing and is to be ignored.

In order to ensure that you are getting the most out of your meditation practice, it is important to eliminate or ignore distractions whenever possible. For example, put pets in another room (or they will steal your lovely meditative energy!), turn off cell phones, and hang a do-not-disturb sign on the door. For distractions that are not so easily put aside, do your best to ignore them. If you find that your mind has wandered off, simply refocus on your mantra.

Let Yourself Sleep

If you find that you are nodding off during meditation, don't worry about it. Don't roughly jerk yourself back to your task. Allow your body to sleep. However, if this is happening every time you meditate, you are most likely not getting enough sleep at night and should consider what changes can be made to your schedule to allow you to get more rest. Adequate sleep is vital to function effectively and feel good.

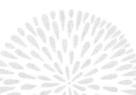
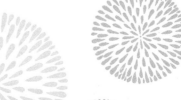

Rely on Your Inner Clock

Your intention should be to meditate for twenty minutes, but you don't want to set an alarm that jolts you awake. Instead, use your inner clock to estimate the amount of time that has passed. If you need help in the beginning, peek with one eye at a nearby watch or clock once in a while. After a few weeks of practice, you'll have an internal sense of time. Using your inner clock and allowing your eyes to stay closed for another few minutes before heading back into the world will allow you to exit your meditation softly rather than abruptly. If you shift too quickly from the meditative state to ordinary waking awareness, you might wind up with a headache.

Using Meditation to Feel Younger and Stay Healthier

You can enjoy the luxury of feeling younger and actually slowing down the aging process when you meditate. There is a developing body of evidence by scientists doing rigorous controlled studies that shows meditation might just be the Fountain of Youth.

One of the first studies on meditating and aging was done in 1982, at which time Dr. Robert Keith Wallace found that a fifty-year-old who had practiced meditation for at least five years actually had a biological age that was no less than twelve years younger![2] Another study, this one from the University of California Los Angeles, suggested that meditators also have less brain shrinkage, which usually happens as we age, as well as better connections between different regions of the brain.[3]

Meditation has also been shown to have other positive effects on health. Studies at the Mind/Body Medical Institute reported a 58 percent decrease in uncomfortable symptoms of PMS and less intensity in hot flashes in women who meditated fifteen to twenty minutes a day. These meditating women also had fewer negative expectations about aging.[4]

In 2007, there was a study called the Shamatha Project, which was done at the Shambhala Mountain Center in Colorado during several three-month retreats.[5] Scientists used monitors connected to the brain and heart waves on meditating subjects at the beginning, middle, and end of each three-month meditation retreat to gather a continuous stream of information. Clifford Saron, a neuroscientist at the Center for Mind and Brain at the University of California, Davis, put together the study. The results were published in 2012. Classic body reactions were detected, of course, such as lower blood pressure, less anxiety, and better cognitive function. The surprise finding came from Elissa Epel, a psychologist from the University of California, San Francisco, who examined the study data and concluded there was a definitive increase in an antiaging process related to telomeres.

What are telomeres? Much like the plastic tips at the ends of shoelaces, telomeres are like caps at either end of every strand of DNA. Telomeres protect your chromosomes, but over time as your cells divide, the telomeres become shorter, and eventually the DNA strands get damaged. This is when your cells age and die. Other factors, including smoking, lack of exercise, stress, a poor diet, or obesity can cause your telomeres to become shorter faster. The meditators in the Shamatha study were shown to have high levels of telomerase, the enzyme that can stop telomeres from getting shorter. Jo Marchant of *The Guardian* reported that Epel explained, "If the increase in telomerase is sustained long enough, it's logical to infer that this group would develop more stable and possibly longer telomeres over time."[6] The implication of this is that meditation could add years to your life. So hop on board the meditation express!

Fill Yourself with Light

I have a meditative-like technique to share with you called the Microcosmic Orbit. It's also known as the circulation of light. This technique comes from the Taoist tradition and is used for cultivating and circulating energy. It sweeps your chi, or personal energy, along the energetic pathways in your body and is central to many Taoist types of exercise, such as T'ai chi and Qigong. It's also called the warm current because the energy it sends throughout your meridians to your chakras is warm. This technique is not a replacement for your daily mantra-based meditation but is a supplement to it, and is especially useful when you're having trouble falling asleep at night.

When you open the Microcosmic Orbit within, you can expand beyond your body and unite with the universal energy field. Try to practice this exercise for about five or ten minutes a day. Your stress level will begin to drop from the very first session, and you'll have more clarity within ten days of practice (especially if you do this exercise daily). One note: try to eliminate or reduce your intake of junk food or food laced with additives and preservatives. A slowly moving Orbit is caused by blockages in the meridians from those impurities. You want your diet to be as healthy as possible for the best results with the Orbit.

Exercise: The Microcosmic Orbit

Take a look at the above diagram to get a clearer idea about how energy flows within your body. You'll see two arrows. The first one, called the governor—or male—channel, begins at the base of the spine and travels up the back, bringing kundalini (primal) energy up the spine. It moves higher than the head and then comes down through the pituitary and pineal gland to the roof of the mouth. This is the yang, or "hot," energy.

The second arrow, called the functional—or female—channel, runs down the front of the body from the tip of the tongue back down to the perineum (the spot that sits right behind your genitals). This is the yin, or "cold," energy.

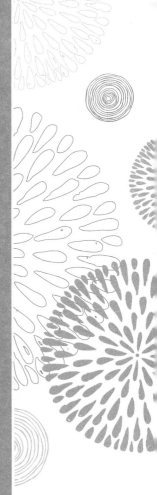

Together, these channels form your Microcosmic Orbit. By learning how to circulate energy and have it flowing smoothly through the Microcosmic Orbit, you will become more conscious of energy and how it moves inside you. Then you will be able to direct and move energy into areas of your body that need healing.

Okay let's gear up and begin. The following steps will show you how to move your energy throughout your body and circulate the orbit. Remember to practice this at a comfortable pace for you.

1 Sit comfortably and close your eyes. (Later when you get more comfortable with this exercise, you can do it standing up or lying down.) Take a deep breath and set your intention to fill yourself with energy and light. Rest your tongue either on the hard palate, the soft part of the roof of your mouth, or behind your upper teeth—whatever position is most comfortable for you.

2 Focus your attention on your lower body or *dan tian*. It's three finger widths below your navel and about a third of the way into your body. Visualize the buildup of light, energy, and warmth until the entire area is filled. Once you progress in your practice and become more attuned to the flow of energy, you may feel the energy as a sense of warmth as it moves through the different stages of the orbit.

3 Imagine warm energy moving from the lower dan tian down toward your tailbone, which is the starting point of the orbit. From there, imagine the energy flowing up your spine, first to the Gate of Life—a dime-size area in the center of the low back at the height of your belly button. From there, proceed up your spinal cord, opening the energy channel.

4 When the warm energy reaches the top of your spine, visualize it heading into your skull to the pineal gland, right in the center of your

head. Pause for a moment or two and then let the energy head down the front of your body.

5 As the warm energy moves down the front of your body, imagine a golden ball of warm energy flowing through the pituitary gland, down the throat and esophagus, into the stomach, and then into the lower dan tian. Let it return to the bottom of your torso, to your perineum, between the anus and the scrotum or vulva, where the orbit began in the area of the tailbone.

6 Continue doing the orbit, circulating the energy, going at a comfortable speed and breathing into any stuck areas. Visualize your channel opening wide.

7 After you have practiced the orbit several times, now imagine the warm energy coming up your spine as you inhale. After holding your breath briefly above the top of the head, exhale as you continue following the orbit down to the dan tian. There, simply relax the energy and let it sink back down to the tailbone area. Each cycle takes one full breath: breathing in up the spine, pausing, and breathing out down the front of the body. Allow your breath to move the ball of energy rather than trying to push it with your will.

Once you feel comfortable circulating energy through your Microcosmic Orbit, you may try this eighth step.

8 The ancient Greeks symbolized the practice of the orbit with the uroboros, which means "serpent biting its tail." When the serpent is biting its tail, it forms a complete circle. As you do the orbit, imagine or feel energy flowing like a conveyor belt or golden serpent through all parts of your body at once. Be easy with yourself while you are learning this new technique.

After you're comfortable doing the orbit, breathing in as you go up the back and exhaling as you go down the front, you can progress to using the following cycle of moving energy as a way to fill yourself with light in order to cope with outside challenges.

1 Feel or imagine a particular upsetting person, event, or situation that is stressful for you now or was in the past. Focus on that person, event, or situation and place it in a box. Visualize that box on the conveyor belt that goes around the orbit.

2 Your orbit may seem to slow down for a while, but don't get discouraged; it will resume normal speed. Keep moving along the orbit until the box and what's in it dissipates. You can also imagine releasing the box into the light when it gets to the pineal gland. If you're visualizing the box and its colors, the orbit itself may look dark or murky for a while; later it will lighten and clear.

3 As the box moves through your Microcosmic Orbit, you may immediately learn the lesson that the situation arose to teach you, or you may have an insight at a later time. It's also possible that nothing will be revealed about that particular situation, but you will see yourself respond differently whenever a similar situation arises. These are all normal responses.

4 When you're done, let your higher consciousness fill the space that opened up when you cleared the stressful matter in the box.

For example, if your father constantly belittled you and called you stupid, you can put your feelings of shame and unworthiness in the box. As the box gets released into the light, the old negative patterns of behavior and thought that you established in order to deal with your father's disempowerment of you won't come back. When faced with challenges, maybe you always thought and acted in ways that resonated with those feelings of unworthiness. Now you can let go of that pattern and get on with your life.

One Final Thought about Meditation

In many ways, meditation is now mainstream, and you can learn different techniques from many sources. However, the meditation you learn from reading about it in a book or online may turn out to be just a basic exercise for reducing stress or relaxing. Meditation is so much more than that. You want to get spiritual benefits as well as physical benefits. Although you can start on your own by doing meditative-like exercises such as the Microcosmic Orbit above, you'll eventually want a qualified instructor to teach you.

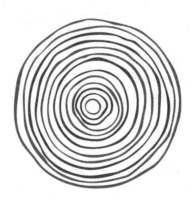

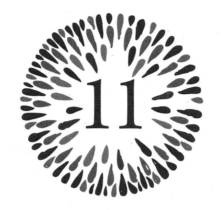

MEET YOUR
SPIRITUAL GUIDES

O nce you start a daily meditation practice, your spiritual guides are not far off. You can tune in to an endless assembly of divine mentors and inner guides who are always waiting in the wings whenever you need them. They're ready to give you their wise counsel, offer instruction for any troubling situations you may face, and give you direction whenever you lose your way.

Unfortunately, these guides aren't visible with ordinary eyesight, although you may have had glimmerings of their presence, such as a whisper in your ear when you most needed help. Maybe you thought it was just your imagination rather than a helping hand in your moment of need. But these guides really do exist and are there for you. All you have to do is ask.

These guides take on a number of different forms—ancestors and deceased loved ones, experts, angels, animals guides, and the Ascended Masters as well as guidance from your own Higher Self.

Let me tell you about each of these guides and how they are there for you along the way.

Ancestors

Most ancient cultures around the world honor their ancestors. Unfortunately, this powerful tradition is nearly lost in the West, along with the wealth of information that these ancestors can provide to us. But if you open your mind, you can receive precious help from these deceased loved ones. It's really a mutual exchange with your relatives: they can help guide you here on earth while you can help guide them into the light of the higher planes.

Usually, your ancestral guide will be a close family member or someone you resonated with, like a favorite uncle or a beloved grandparent. This ancestor could also be someone you didn't know when they were alive but is part of your family lineage. All of us have relatives, either recently departed or long gone, who are ready to be of service, no matter how imperfect their life might have seemed.

My grandfather was a drinker who frequently lost his job as a firefighter, but his final illness, which was painful and frightening for him, may have helped him clean up his act. Now he serves as my guide whenever I get lost, either hiking or driving; he's really good at giving directions. Seek out your deceased loved ones who can help you in particular areas of your life. Maybe one was an artist who can offer you guidance in your creative projects or a businessman who can help you straighten out your finances.

You can pick up an abundance of knowledge and insight when you start digging into your familial roots. For example, I was happy to learn that my grandmother from Portugal was a healer. I love connecting on a regular basis to my grandmother to support my healing lineage.

If you know where your ancestors came from and around what time period they lived in, you can look up what happened in history during that time and place. Your ancestors may have lived through war or natural disasters. Perhaps they escaped from religious persecution by sailing to the New World. Or maybe they were members of an indigenous tribe in the Americas that was decimated by Europeans. Conversely, they could have been the people who started the war, led the religious persecution, or were the conquerors. The deep wounding from those painful memories can carry over for generations.

Learning your family history can help you to understand some parts of yourself that may not have been clear before. Although it may seem illogical or even absurd, what your ancestor experienced can indeed affect you today. Their bad mojo can be passed down to you, and you can indeed suffer for the sins of your ancestors. Try to forgive any ancestor who did wrong. You can pray for the deceased to heal so dysfunctional family patterns can be dissolved and not affect future generations. Rituals or ceremonies or prayers can help heal your ancestors while also helping you to heal at the same time.

You may also have strong roots with your ancestral guides from a previous life. One of my Jewish friends from New York has an affinity for the foothills of the Himalayas—the only location that feels like home to her. She undoubtedly has roots in India from past lives, so she turns to those ancestors for guidance. At my workshops, I frequently see someone reflect an image from an ancestor that holds strong roots or important lessons for that person.

It's not necessary to believe in past lifetimes to access your ancestral guides. My experience is that we are having simultaneous experiences on various planes, so just keep your mind open. Then you can decide whether to accept, reject, or change your mind about this information.

Exercise: Connecting with Your Ancestor

Your parents or grandparents are the most likely to come to your aid, but you could receive help from any member of your family tree using this method. Be sure to keep your intentions positive so you only link with positive energies.

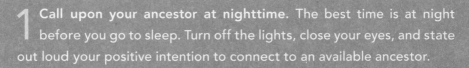

1 **Call upon your ancestor at nighttime.** The best time is at night before you go to sleep. Turn off the lights, close your eyes, and state out loud your positive intention to connect to an available ancestor.

2 **Choose the ancestor you resonate with the most.** This is often the first one who comes to mind.

3 **Picture your ancestor in whatever form you like.** You may remember your grandfather as a grumpy old man, but you have a picture of him as a handsome young guy in his wedding photo. Even though you don't remember him that way (you weren't even born yet), you can use that image to connect with him if you wish.

4 **Ask for something specific.** Ask this ancestor for help with a real problem or specific family issue. You may encounter this ancestral guide later in your dreams or suddenly come up with a solution to your problem after your meditation.

Remember, your ancestors and all of your guides want to help you, but they must be *specifically asked*. Whatever information you get from them also depends on how well connected they are to Source. My darling aunt is great with family issues, but I'd never ask her for help in healing somebody.

Experts

You can also seek help from any professionals or experts in the field who have passed on. If I'm wearing my healer hat, I call upon the great healers of history, including Jesus. When I was in Brazil working with John of God, a noted healer and psychic surgeon, I "met" quite a few deceased physicians and surgeons who guide him, and some of them remained available to me after I returned. I often feel them working through me.

If you're a writer having trouble developing a character or coming up with a great love scene, you could call upon writers you admire to help—maybe Jackie Collins can help you add more sizzle. If you're a student facing a difficult psychology exam, you can seek out Sigmund Freud or Carl Jung to help you understand the material.

Calling on Expert Guides

Please treat your expert guides with humility and respect, just as you would a living professional. Think of what it is you need help with and set an intention for a guide from this field to join you. Visualize a ball of light surrounding you—a shield that allows only that which is for your highest good to come through. Humbly ask for help and listen within to "hear" their advice and instruction. And remember to thank them. This gesture of gratitude will continue to build a strong bond between you and your guides.

Angels

When engaging in energy healing, you most definitely want to enlist angels as your guiding lights. They are talented healers and act as a conduit between you and the universal energy field, and they form a bridge between you and your clients. They help you connect to your own divine energy and your Higher Self as well as to the divine energies of Source. Angels bring messages from your Higher Self and sometimes from forces beyond your knowledge. When angels are around, good things are bound to happen, including healing physical ailments, emotional problems, and spiritual concerns.

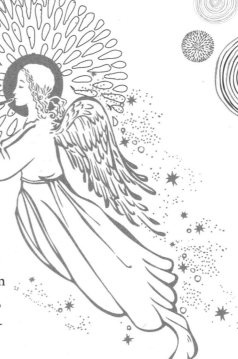

Calling on Angels

In order to call upon your angels for help, all you need to do is set an intention; don't worry if you don't sense them—they're there. What's really important is knowing that you need to request their help. Just like all the other guides, angels don't volunteer their services unasked for.

You have personal guardian angels, and just above them are the archangels. I'd start by asking your guardian angel to help you. You'll establish a stronger angelic energy connection when you choose a name for your guardian angel. You can come up with a visual image and a specific gender as well. Now, all you have to do is ask for a sign that your guardian angel is with you. Talk to your angel, either silently or out loud, and ask for specific signs. Keep asking until you actually get one.

As I've said before, always thank your guides when they come to your aid. They appreciate the gratitude, and it's a great way to strengthen your connection with them. The more you call upon them, the brighter your energy field will be, thus attracting them into your life even more. I usually contact my angel guides before meditating in the morning and again before going to sleep, but you can call upon your angels as often as you need them and continue to send them love and gratitude. You can easily connect with your angels in your sixth chakra, since your third eye is the best point for accessing angelic energy. It's here you can conceive of your life's plan and start moving in that direction.

If you feel that you've made a mess of your life, no need to worry. This won't scare the angels away. They only see you in your perfection, even if you're not living perfectly. Angels never judge, no matter what. That's what makes them tops in the book of spiritual guides. They have a high vibration of unconditional love!

Animal Guides

There's another group of guides that you can always rely on—those from the animal kingdom! Animal guides can be of great help when it comes to clearing your chakras and connecting to the energy you need to heal yourself and others. Animals are wiser than we are, as they know how to live in harmony with the earth, and they utilize all their senses, far beyond what any human can do.

Each animal carries its own knowledge and powers. Land-based animals connect you to your intuition and consciousness. The bear, for example, is the Primal Mother and teaches the value of introspection, since bears know when to be alone and hibernate. Those swimming in the water aid you in acknowledging any thoughts or actions that are hidden from your awareness. For example, fish of the deep oceans are considered the sacred messengers of ancient wisdom, and it is said that dreaming of a porpoise will reveal your true gift, while whales can align you with your inner voice and help you to sing your individual song. Those flying high in the air connect you to higher knowledge. The eagle, for instance, brings you messages from the center of the sun and transports your prayers up to the realm of the creator. Insects teach you to work in harmony with nature. In particular, we are slowly learning the importance of bees (hopefully not too late), which play a key role in pollination, symbolize fertility, and are the keepers of hidden wisdom.

An animal guide doesn't even have to be a real animal. A dragon can show up in your dream, breathing fire to annihilate some of your fear. If the mythical phoenix appears at any time, be ready for a major transformation or a great renewal of some sort. Unicorns or mermaids can also send you guidance.

Calling on Animal Guides

To communicate with animal guides, you'll need a great deal of patience and practice. One way to encounter your animal guide is to go on a spirit guide walk somewhere in nature and stay open to any sign or symbol along the way that feels right in your heart. The bird feather that flutters to the ground in front of you, the snake that wriggles past you as you walk in the woods, the way your horse shies away from someone you thought was trustworthy— over and over again you receive messages from your animal guides.

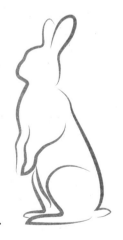

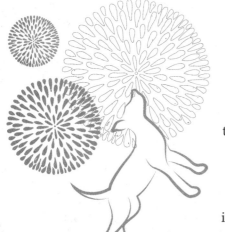

Invite the animals you think you might be connected to, and then wait to see which ones actually show up. When you meditate, you can set an intention and ask the name of your totem animals. These are the animals connected to each of your chakras as they ascend up the spine. As you bring your attention to each chakra, humbly request to feel or see that chakra's animal. You will be able to gather a lot of information about the energetic state of your chakras by seeing what animal shows up. A terrified rabbit in your base chakra is looking for more stability and security. A wounded elephant in your heart is a large hurt that needs healing. A soaring eagle in your third eye can mean you are ready to ascend to higher planes. Mentally feed those animals who seem hungry with your love and compassion. And remember, you have to ask for the animal's help.

Ascended Masters

It may seem like a wild leap to go from a bouncing bunny or slithering snake to the hierarchy of the Great White Brotherhood, but in fact the Ascended Masters can also be called upon as spirit guides.

Who are the Ascended Masters? Ascended Masters were like you and me once upon a time, but through many lifetimes of inner work they have united with their Higher Self and gained ascension. This means they have gone through the initiatory process of spiritual transformation, have taken the sixth initiation, and can dwell on the sixth dimension fully merged with their mighty I AM presence. Ascended Masters have invaluable wisdom to share with you because they have attained the highest goal and are here to help.

There are many spiritual masters on higher and higher levels of the Great White Brotherhood. (Note: The *white* refers to the pure white light, not skin color, and *brotherhood* includes both males and females.) You may have heard them referred to as the Great Universal Brotherhood, the Lords of the Flame or the Lords of Light. A spiritual master who has taken the ninth initiation (the highest on the three-dimensional planet of Earth) is a Lord of the World.

What exactly have these beings attained? Their enlightenment, which started like yours as moments of spiritual insight, has become a deep fundamental state of being in them. In Buddhism, a bodhisattva is someone who understands the way to liberation. Someone in buddhahood experiences the fullness of awakening, where wisdom, compassion, and skill are fully present. Hindus say someone has attained *moksha* (liberation, freedom from all passions and desires), while a fully awakened one has *sat-chit-ananda* (complete truth, knowledge, and bliss). They are in *sahaj samadhi*—with each and every breath, they are going in and out of the highest state of consciousness that can be attained while in a body. So being enlightened, fully awakened, means you go beyond any form of an external God and completely know your own Higher Self—it's an arc that goes from worshipping a being like Jesus to merging into the Christ light yourself.

This is the world of the mystics—those initiates who have experienced a state of higher consciousness. Fully realized mystics have been the starting point of every religion, and every religion has a mystic center: Gnostics in Christianity, Kabbalists in Judaism, Sufis in Islam, and the saints and sages of Hinduism and Buddhism. This central core is the "secret" knowledge of being One with God. It can be called the *Secret Doctrine* or *Teachings of the Temple*, but it is the same truth in every religion and culture, presented as different versions of the sacred trinity: creator, preserver, destroyer (Brahma, Vishnu, Shiva); spirit, soul, matter; father, mother, son; father, son, and holy spirit.

Throughout all of recorded history, and undoubtedly before that, these Ascended Masters have been available to those who connect to the threefold flame anchored in their spiritual heart and are dedicated to serving the Light. Your threefold flame is made of the blue plume (the will and

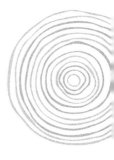

power of God), the yellow plume (the right use of wisdom and discrimination), and the pink plume (love and compassion). When the three plumes of the flame are in balance within the heart, power is tempered by love, and love is filled with wisdom.

The risen Jesus is called Sananda on the inner planes. Along with Archangel Uriel, he works on bringing brotherhood, peace, the concept of service, and freedom to all people. He can guide you to a deeper understanding of the power of unconditional love and help you to do more loving actions in your life. Lady Nada is the Ascended Master who incarnated as John the Baptist's mother, Elizabeth. She is the leader of the ray of service. Her name Nada, translates as the "voice of the silence," and she is the one to call upon if you are interested in sound healing. Along with Lady Masters Pallas Athena (the Goddess of Truth) and Kuan Yin, these masters are helping to balance out the masculine and feminine energies on earth.

The Western Ascended Masters include Mother Mary, who is a protector of women and children as well as a helper with healing. In an earlier incarnation in ancient Egypt, she was Isis, who taught initiates the Mysteries. Also in Egypt was Hermes Trismegistus, called the scribe of the gods. He was a noted theologian, sage, and patron of esoteric scholars and alchemists—seeking the reconciliation of opposites through transformation. If you called on him, he would help you either to untangle the deep questions you may have puzzled over in philosophy or to understand the hidden mysteries.

While alchemists tried to change the base metal of lead into gold, the masters are here to help us change our consciousness through self-transformation. Master Kuthumi, El Morya, Djwhal Khul (the Tibetan), and Saint Germain all work together to bring about our enlightenment.

Exercise: The Violet Flame

Count Saint Germain, the Ascended Master of the Aquarian Age (in charge of America), gifted those of us on earth with the transmuting power of the Violet Flame. This is a powerful way to work with energy. It can bring forth courage from fear, love from hatred, and peace from anxiety. You can use the Violet Flame to transmute difficult aspects of your karma and to help others do the same. You can even use the Violet Flame to lend your energy to transmuting troubles in the world.

The Violet Flame is a prayer through which you invoke your I AM presence (your Higher Self) to transmute any situation into the energy of divine light. Use it to get unstuck from a victim mentality and to dissipate fear, negativity, or energetic blockages. You don't ask for a particular solution; you simply allow for the divine plan to bring things into harmony.

Bring your attention to your heart chakra and visualize a violet flame there as you *feel* the words of the prayer. The flame is not hot like a fire; it is simply the energetic manifestation of the violet ray. Say the following prayer over and over again until you feel a shift in energy:

My beloved, divine I AM presence, blaze in, through, and around me your Violet Flame of Transmutation. I now call forth the full and complete power of the Violet Flame to transmute [any negativity] (you could name shame, anger, self-hatred, lack, or a personal limitation of any kind, like ill health) *that resides within me in its cause, core, etheric records, memories, and effects. With love and forgiveness, I blaze forth the Violet Flame throughout my entire energy field. I humbly ask my mighty I AM presence to fill me with the golden light of Spirit in infinite light, love, abundance, and health. And so it is.*

You have now burned up your negativity in the violet flame and transformed it into the light of Spirit.

In the Indian tradition, there are great saints and avatars (incarnations of God, not symbols used in video gaming). Babaji, the immortal

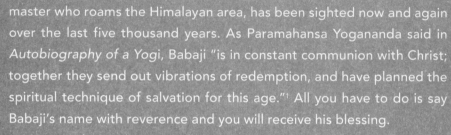

master who roams the Himalayan area, has been sighted now and again over the last five thousand years. As Paramahansa Yogananda said in *Autobiography of a Yogi*, Babaji "is in constant communion with Christ; together they send out vibrations of redemption, and have planned the spiritual technique of salvation for this age."[1] All you have to do is say Babaji's name with reverence and you will receive his blessing.

More modern Indian saints have many devotees from the West, including Meher Baba, Ramana Maharshi (who taught his devotees self-inquiry with the question, who am I?), and Ramakrishna (who worshipped the goddess Kali and can connect you to the divine mother). Those who are attracted to Buddhism can ask guidance of Kuan Yin (the goddess of mercy), the Tibetan saint Milarepa, and Maitreya (the head of the Great Universal Brotherhood). Another Tibetan is Lady Master Leto, who is the twin flame of Djwhal Khul and is closely connected to Saint Germain. She is an especially important connection for those who need help raising indigo and crystal children, who are light workers and can have psychic and telepathic abilities for healing the world.

These are only some of the Ascended Masters you can call upon as spiritual guides. They are unified with the Mind of God and embody unconditional love. They serve as the guardians of all humanity.

Your Higher Self

Finally, the time has come to meet the most important of all inner guides—*you*. Not just you, but the real, authentic, and awesome you—the one living deep inside under all the layers of doubt, fear, insecurity, and negativity. The one who is confident and has it all together. The one who doesn't pay attention to any distractions or temptations on the outside. This pure and real you is your Higher Self—your most powerful and reliable source of accurate information. To hear it, you have to listen and follow your "gut feelings" because these are your best channel for intuitive messages. Your Higher Self is very important when you're working to heal someone else. Your Higher Self can attune to the Higher Self of the other person, and when you listen with the advanced hearing of your Higher Self, you will learn valuable information that will help in your healing session.

Multiple Types of Consciousness

There are four different types of consciousness: waking, dreaming, sleeping, and meditating. In your normal waking consciousness, you basically get information from your five senses: taste, touch, sight, hearing, and smell. This is where your rational thinking mind is most comfortable. Here, your mind develops certain beliefs, builds protective walls against pain and suffering, and blames others for anything that goes wrong in life. It's the only reality many people know and accept.

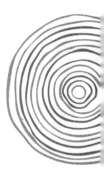

The second state of consciousness is where your subconscious creates dreams to clear out stressful thoughts. Sometimes, your guides can send you messages through your dreams.

In the third type of consciousness, you are asleep—to everything!

The fourth and highest type of consciousness, the meditative state, happens when you *wake up*, not only from your sleep and dreams but also from your ordinary state of awareness. It is here that you move beyond the ordinary and take the leap into personal growth and higher states of consciousness, where you start to take responsibility for your life. It sometimes takes a fair amount of self-healing work to experience this level of consciousness. But when you do, you'll begin to realize that material things, like a brand-new wardrobe or a big promotion, aren't going to make you feel more secure. You'll start to embrace your Higher Self and ultimately discover that all wisdom lies within you.

When you are fully aligned and balanced, you'll have more energy and vitality, more stable health, and a better ability to receive healing. Your thoughts will become deeper, with a real understanding of your spiritual nature. You'll be happy, joyful, passionate, peaceful, and in harmony with your life. Your heart will be open and filled with love, and your creativity will sparkle.

Connecting with Your Higher Self

The very best way to get in touch with your Higher Self is through meditation. When your mind calms down and your thoughts grow silent, you will be able to hear the voice of your Higher Self. Meditation will also quiet your emotions and all the unresolved feelings that disturb your inner peace. Meditation lets you sit in your heart, where the Higher Self can be heard most clearly.

After you have done twenty minutes of mantra-based meditation or before you go to sleep at night, imagine your Higher Self is around two or three feet above the top of your head, in your eighth chakra. Invite your Higher Self to enter your body so you can feel its presence. Welcome it and ask for your connection to grow in strength. Imagine your vibratory rate increasing. Anything you feel is going to be unique to you, not only over time, but also every time you complete this practice. Your experience of it can shift from moment to moment, but you may also experience certain energies in the same way every time. For example, dark energy may always make you feel a heaviness at the base of your neck, whereas light energy may feel like effervescent bubbles inside of you. Most, but not everyone, gets bodily sensations. You may feel your shoulders opening and your chest expanding in the light, and closing and contracting in the dark. Personally, I get two different kinds of goose bumps that differentiate light and dark energies.

Ask your Higher Self for whatever you feel you need. You can ask to send energy to those you love. Always thank your Higher Self for any message.

You can develop a stronger connection with your Higher Self by journaling your feelings, insights, and dreams. Write down any questions you may have for your Higher Self. Keep writing down your dreams too. This is a great way to understand and interpret the messages brought to you. Be aware of any hunches, whispers, or gut feelings that you may have ignored in the past. They could hold valuable information that could help you avoid negative situations.

Next we're going to examine another great tool to help you read the twists and turns of human energy: mind/body types and their defense mechanisms.

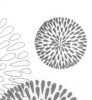

MIND/BODY TYPES

Our human energy field encounters many outside forces that can shape and reshape the field. Mind/body types show us the ways energy gets twisted during our early years (from the womb to around the age of seven) into body shapes and psychological defense mechanisms that we use to protect ourselves. If I could only teach you two things in life, I would teach you how to meditate and how to identify and work with mind/body types and then send you back to your life—to the corporate world, the nonprofit world, the parenting world, wherever. If you learn and practice those two tools, you will really be in command of your life.

Your chakras develop as your body grows from an infant to an adult. Naturally, an immature body will have immature chakras. The chakras develop according to the psychological patterns you learn. We all tend to block or bury our feelings in reaction to traumas and generally unpleasant experiences. When we do that, we stop the flow of energy in that area, which affects the chakra's development. When a chakra is closed and spinning counterclockwise, you send your energy outward into the world. Psychologists call this *projection*. What is happening is that you are creating a belief system about the reality of the world that is really nothing more than your projection.

For instance, a mom is diagnosed with a difficult disease after her son is born, and she spends a long time in the hospital away from the child. The infant misses his mother and feels rejected by her. He closes his heart chakra to protect himself from the pain of the perceived rejection. He may grow up believing the world is unloving, while in fact this belief is based in his own feelings that he is projecting onto the world.

Whenever you have a frightening or painful experience that you block out, you are also blocking out the positive emotions. That chakra will eventually become distorted, clog with energy that has turned stagnant, start spinning in the wrong way, or stop moving altogether, and if not corrected, this can lead to a physical disease or problem. Note that the way a chakra is spinning is from the perspective of someone looking at you, not you looking from the inside out. Most people have a few chakras out of sync unless they've done a lot of personal work.

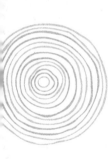

I teach mind/body types in energy medicine because they are such a clear expression of how the emotions impact the physical body and the chakras. Once you've mastered identifying with mind/body types, you can look at people and have a good idea about what sort of traumas they went through early in life and to what extent the defense mechanisms they learned at that time are still with them. The energy of the emotions actually created the physical appearance of the body. For those who are studying energy medicine, it is wonderful shorthand for getting a quick read on someone you will be working with. If you use this system to examine yourself, you can learn which areas you need to work on so you can heal old traumas and learn to express yourself in a more authentic way.

What Do Mind/Body Types Stem From?

Mind/body types (sometimes called characterology) are a system that, most recently, grew out of psychology, when psychology married bodywork. This

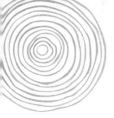

happened in the late 1940s and early 1950s with Alexander Lowen, but I have found the same type of work in the Greek classics, in East Indian Ayurveda, in all cultures in which people figured out that some people have bodies that look a certain way because of something that happened to them when they were little.

In the 1950s, Alexander Lowen popularized bioenergetic analysis, a type of mind/body psychotherapy, with his colleague John Pierrakos. In Lowen's 1975 book, *Bioenergetics*, he used terms that we still use today, which were the Freudian definitions of personality disorders that were accepted by the psychiatric profession. Later, John's wife, Eva Pierrakos, a spiritual teacher, added the energetic and spiritual aspects to each of the five character structures.

The Mind/Body Types in Depth

The terms for the five character types, which are also known as defense mechanisms, are:

- **Schizoid:** This comes from the word *schizophrenia* and indicates people who are "out of touch" with external reality and not grounded, not that they are schizophrenic.

- **Oral:** This refers to infancy when one clings to others and needs to be held. These people have trouble being independent, since their underlying feeling is that of deprivation.

- **Psychopath:** Again, this does not mean these people are psychopaths but rather that most of their energy is held in the head.

- **Masochist:** This not a reference to masochism as it is usually defined. This refers to people who complain but remain submissive. These people block their feelings of superiority and hostility so they won't explode.

- **Rigid:** As it sounds, these people are stiff with pride, but it is a defensive posture to protect against the fear of being controlled.

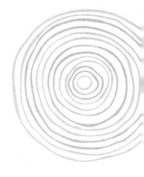

I have found through decades of energy healing that at heart, our problems are always based on a distorted belief about ourselves. Our self-loathing shows itself in different ways through the different mind/body structures. Please realize that what constitutes a trauma for one infant or child may have no impact on another. It all depends on what life lessons that soul has incarnated in order to learn.

To use mind/body types in healing yourself, you want to find out which defense mechanisms you use, although you have to remember they are not who you are; they are who you are *not*. You also want to find out when you use them. You may start to realize, *Wow, anytime that particular thing happens, I go into this mind/body type.* Once you understand your habitual reaction, you can gradually change it.

Let's go into each of the mind/body types in depth.

Schizoid

The schizoid character is always discussed first because it develops first in time, which is in the womb or at birth. So many things can happen then, but the most common scenario is a hostile mother. Your mother could be living through a war, could be a refugee or prisoner, could live through a natural disaster or a bitter divorce, could be grieving a parent's death during this time, or she could be going through a problem pregnancy or a difficult birth. Maybe she was told labor and birth were horrible experiences, and she was afraid.

A "hostile" mother simply means that at some point during pregnancy or the birth, she felt angry, which the infant perceives as: *I'm not wanted. This is high risk. I've got to get out of here.* As a fetus and infant, your chakras are not well developed, nor is your nervous system. So you develop a particular coping mechanism, which in this case is to get the hell out of Dodge—split off from the external world and from scary internal feelings by going back into the safe world of Spirit.

This defense works well when you're young but is probably holding you back as an adult. When something or someone challenges you, do you leave your body? Why would you keep using an outdated coping mechanism? Because it worked back then? If you can leave your body quite easily and you experience a lot of fear and anxiety, you may very well still be using the schizoid defense.

Generally, we don't use only one of the defense mechanisms; most of us are a combination of several, and have one or two that are predominant in our makeup.

So let's get back to infancy. Maybe mom is afraid of her partner or has been abandoned to face pregnancy alone. Maybe she never really wanted children but is pressured by her religion or her own morals to not have an abortion. So what is the first thing the child is going to feel? Rejection. The schizoid doesn't feel that he has the right to exist, so it's too risky to stick around.

When a person with a schizoid defense mechanism is faced with a threatening situation, or at least perceives it as threatening, he contracts energetically and draws back into the safety of the spirit world. It becomes habitual to leave the physical body by splitting off his consciousness and twisting it so most of the energy can escape from the top of the head. This weakens the person's energy field and actually makes it easier for others to penetrate, reaffirming his feeling that the world is not a safe place.

I've noticed that those who develop a strong schizoid character have often had past lives that were traumatic, either from physical pain, death from torture, or other severe trauma. They come into this life reluctantly, expecting the world to be hostile, and so wind up choosing parents who make this a reality.

What do schizoids look like? Usually, they will have a long body with weak or hyperextended joints, cold hands and feet, and possibly a twist in the spine from avoiding physical reality and flying out of the body. When they are in their defense mechanism, they may look like they are staring into space or simply not present. They are ungrounded and might be called flaky. When you try to relate to them, they will withdraw or will speak intellectually, without much emotional context. Their most common physical problems stem from having accidents because they are ungrounded.

The schizoid defense mechanism works like this: *I almost died early in life, maybe at birth. I'm certainly going to die. I don't want to be destroyed. My solution is to reject you so you can't reject me and spin me out into an existential terror.* My student Betsy is a good example. She is biracial. Betsy's mother was rejected by

her family for having a relationship with someone of a different race, and they rejected the child she carried as well. Her mother had previously suffered several miscarriages, so she was nervous all throughout the pregnancy. When Betsy was born, her mother had to stay in the hospital for several weeks to receive blood transfusions, so even as a newborn, Betsy felt abandoned. All these difficult experiences in the womb and at birth were the root of her schizoid defense mechanism. When Betsy is under pressure, she tends to stop paying attention to her surroundings, which makes it hard for her to keep a job. Betsy has learned the triggers that bring on this defense mechanism and takes steps to correct herself when she feels this behavior coming on.

Your body grows from the blueprint of your energy field, which can get distorted from early traumatic experiences. When you become aware of your defense mechanisms—and there is usually more than one—just focusing your attention on them helps you to stop using that particular mechanism.

Often, those with the schizoid defense mechanism are very spiritual, with a deep connection to their life purpose and understanding of the meaning of life. Their sixth level of the field, the celestial body, will be very strong, filled with bright colors. They can bring spirituality into the lives of others. Their life lesson becomes facing the rage and terror inside so they can fully manifest their spirituality and creativity in the world. Their imbalance is mainly in the lower chakras, since they take in less energy than they give out. Many chakras may be spinning counterclockwise. The second, third, sixth, and seventh chakras, when they are open, may be asymmetrical or not balanced in the way they function.

In order to heal, schizoids have to learn to stay grounded and to actually feel their emotions, no matter how intense, and release them. Any means of self-expression, such as writing or journaling, can help manifest their spirituality in the physical world. They have to allow for self-love and to live according to the truth of who they are. Bit by bit, they can reintegrate themselves by paying attention to self-care of the body and reclaiming their right to be here and to participate in life.

To give you an idea of what each type looks like, I'm going to give you some examples of celebrities who fit each type. Pop culture seems to be our common meeting ground these days, so you probably will recognize the people you see all the time in film and on television and in celebrity magazines. The classic schizoid is Diane Keaton as Annie Hall in Woody Allen's movie *Annie Hall*. She's spacey, out-of-body, with loose joints. Another schizoid is the character Carrie that Claire Danes plays on the television series *Homeland*. Jim Carrey also has that elongated body and often takes roles in which he plays a schizoid character type.

Oral

Between the first six weeks of life and up to a year old, during the normal time frame for breastfeeding, the oral character just wasn't fed or cared for enough because of either physical or emotional abandonment by the mother. This is a life-threatening situation. If Mom can't produce enough breast milk, or if she's busy with other young children, or she's got you on a feeding schedule and lets you cry when you're hungry if it isn't the "right time" yet, you will probably manifest the oral defense mechanism.

Suckling, either at the breast or bottle, lets the infant bond with the mother. If for whatever reason this bonding with the mother is skipped or cut short, the child may never feel the comfort and security needed to develop in a healthy manner.

It may not be your mom's fault, not intentionally, but that doesn't stop you from feeling her rejection. You are hungry and aren't being fed, so you stifle the feeling of hunger, of need. You may be too scared about asking for whatever you need, because your experience is that it won't be given. You can never get "enough." So you respond to this early trauma by clinging to others and sucking the energy from them. This is the birth of the energy vampire, the drama queen, who you will learn about in the next chapter. The thinking is, *There's not enough for me, so I need to fill up on energy I take from you*. Hopefully, this defense comes up only when you are threatened in some way and is not your habitual stance in life. Or you might turn greedy, needing to hold on to whatever you can. Orals want the right to be fulfilled, to be nurtured. Their biggest problem is fatigue; they seem too tired to stand up for themselves. Codependency is so much easier, with the thought process being, *Let someone else take care of me.*

All orals want is to be nurtured, so we tend to see them as needy and incapable of acting on their own. In fact, they are great at manipulating others. Their voice is low, and they ask many questions; you have to listen carefully to get what they are saying. Their double-bind problem is that if they have to ask for it, it's not really love; but if they don't ask, they won't get it. So what does their mask say? *I don't need you.* In reality, everything about them shouts neediness.

As would be expected, the oral character takes refuge in eating, talking, and smoking. In past lives, orals may have starved to death or been through a famine. They choose to be born to heal their expectation of abandonment and rejection, to heal their belief that they cannot take care of themselves. They may suffer from passivity and fatigue, since they always seem to be in need of nourishment.

The oral character's main energy is in the head, with the sixth and seventh chakras being the most open, which explains their preference for intellectual and verbal pursuits rather than for physical movement.

Physically, people with the oral character may have flaccid muscles and a collapsed chest. Their shoulders slump down. They always seem to lack energy and tire easily or feel depressed. Their legs are weak, with fallen arches in the feet. Or they may look immature. Their eyes have that puppy-dog pleading look. Their general energy is low because all their energy is usually in the head. Anne Hathaway as Fantine in *Les Miserables* is a perfect example of the oral character. Jake Gyllenhaal has the oral's eyes in the film *Brokeback Mountain*, pleading with you to love him.

Energetically, orals try to attach cords from their third chakra to others in order to draw out their energy. Or they may suck energy through eye contact, which establishes bioplasmic streamers. Their chakras don't reach a normal size because they are using so much energy to draw from others. Their field stays weak and can't be filled from inside, so they are stuck relying on others. Since it's not very pleasant to be around oral characters, their interactions with others often lead to more rejection, what they see as more proof that they don't have the right to get their needs met.

Frequently, orals engage in service to others, hoping to earn the right to receive—this is service from a place of neediness and leads to more exhaustion. Their life lesson is to stop being a victim and experience being completely filled up by themselves, to realize their own power to take care of themselves. Then they can give to others from a place of fullness, not neediness. Oral characters need to work on releasing their grief about not getting enough good mothering as a child. They can connect to the earth, the Great Mother, who is always available. Getting more grounded will charge their chakras and bring in more energy, and then they can direct their immense ability to love at themselves and nourish themselves before giving to others.

Psychopath

The psychopathic defense mechanism develops between the ages of eighteen months and four years as the child is forming an unspoken alliance with the parent of the opposite sex. So if it's a girl, Daddy (or a father figure) sides with her and they gang up against the mother. In her mind, the little girl is Daddy's partner. She might even say, "I'm going to marry Daddy." Maybe her mom and dad aren't getting along with each other, but they have no trouble getting along with their child, who then starts fantasizing that Daddy is all hers. Of course, that isn't usually how it really is, so next comes the feeling of betrayal.

The defense mechanism that develops at this stage will be a controlling attitude that says, "My way or the highway." Psychopaths need to win, and to look good. If they feel defeated, they will lie to protect themselves. They are a lot like the oral character in being needy and insecure, but they cover it up with an ideal image that can admit no wrong. They make themselves appear as large and aggressive as possible with the idea that they can somehow control the situation. Psychopaths need to be able to trust, but the sting of betrayal lingers. So they hide behind the mask of *I'm right and you're wrong*.

It's easy to tell who the psychopaths are. This is generally the most intimidating and controlling character, with a great ability to communicate and perform. Actors, singers, lawyers, and politicians all have some aspects of this character structure. James Gandolfini as Tony Soprano in *The Sopranos* is a classic psychopath.

In previous lifetimes psychopaths may have been warriors who fought for a good cause; they were the "good" ones winning over the "bad" ones. But they were betrayed, possibly by those they trusted the most. Now they believe that no one is trustworthy. The world is scary and they need to control it, so they try to dominate others in any way—bullying, manipulating, seducing, overpowering, and lying. They are aggressive and thus attract aggression in return; life truly becomes a battleground.

Psychopaths are attractive, with a commanding and confident appearance. They may be larger up top than in the lower body, since they pull their energy up and out, and their upper half is therefore more energetically charged than the lower. Sometimes this character structure is called displaced because of this displacement of energy. Although this defense mechanism forms during the time the third chakra is developing, the displacement of energy focuses on the fifth chakra, which is why they can be such great communicators, with eloquent powers of seduction. While the upper chakras can be open, the feeling centers tend to be closed. The first and second chakras, in particular, are depleted by the way the energy is displaced, so psychopaths may be ungrounded as well as undercharged sexually. Their seductive powers don't lead to intimate and lasting relationships, since they are always expecting to be betrayed by their partner, and sex is seen more as a conquest than shared pleasure.

The displaced energy may create an upper body that has broad shoulders and narrow hips, with a cold, tight pelvis. The legs may be weak. Their eyes are compelling, and their energy is hyperactive followed by collapse after doing too much. They may throw themselves at people and situations, and then collapse with exhaustion. Generally, however, their health will be good, with the exception of problems in the back or joints. They are also more likely to have heart attacks since they closed their heart chakra down from the pain of so much betrayal.

The life lesson for psychopaths is to overcome their need to control others and learn to trust them as well as to learn to trust themselves. Healing comes about when they feel safe, when they can make a mistake and it's okay to do so because they know they are human. They realize they don't always have to win or be special but can feel like it's enough to be part of humanity. When the psychopathic defense mechanism is released, these people have a lot of integrity and can bring truth, valor, and determination into life.

Then there are closet psychopaths—people who smile at you while throwing their energy up their back, over their head, and out the third eye right at you. This is a kill-or-be-killed behavior. It is a defense mechanism for people who were disempowered at some time in their lives. It's what I would do as a young lawyer: I'd enter the courtroom in a short skirt and sweetly con the judge and the other lawyer, and then I'd nail them. Often, those who are very gifted as speakers, performers, actors, and lawyers will have some psychopathic energy because they need to be able to call up that energy and send it out to their audience.

Remember that defense mechanisms are built on a foundation of fear. If you were traumatized as an infant or young child and get scared that you're about to be hurt or trapped or vulnerable in some way, you will find a protective way to defend yourself. If I call someone a psychopath, all I'm saying is that the person uses the psychopath defense mechanism when feeling threatened or pushed. We all go to our habitual defense mechanism when we're backed up against a wall. Don't be embarrassed when one of your defense mechanisms shows up; just note it—*Ah, there's the old psychopath coming out again!*

Masochist

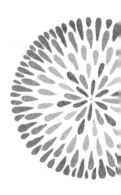

The masochistic defense mechanism begins in children when they are starting to become independent between the ages of two and four (same as psychopaths), and are dominated by a parent who pressures them about when and what they are allowed to eat, or exerts control over bodily functions or what clothes to wear or how they do their hair. They might exert so much control over the children that they even finish their sentences and allow them no personal space.

Energetically, the children may feel like they're being crushed—they aren't being allowed to develop any autonomy—and there's an explosion building up inside that can't get out. The parent squashed the children's self-expression and then the children were made to feel guilty about it. There is no resort but submission. The children are humiliated and hold inside all their feelings, real self-expression, and creativity in order to get the parent's approval.

What happens? These children feel defeated and trapped, full of tension. They comply because they want parental approval, but they wind up fearing their own anger. This is the double bind: *If I get angry, I'll be humiliated. If I don't get angry, I'll be humiliated.* Their greatest fear is being humiliated. So what do they do? They hurt themselves before anyone else can hurt them. Instead of outwardly expressing the anger from continually not honoring their own self, these children turn it inward and develop a harsh inner critic.

Eventually, we all parent ourselves, treating ourselves the same way our parents treated us. If we had a lot of pressure to be a certain way growing up, we then put a lot of pressure on ourselves internally. Passive-aggressive complaining or whining is an unconscious way to provoke anger in others so masochists have permission to get angry in return. In other words, this mind/body type is dependent on others for self-expression.

It is possible that these masochists had many lifetimes of being suppressed and controlled by others, perhaps being imprisoned or enslaved or subjected to the rules of religious or political groups. This time they chose parents who became their captors. Because of the way they have learned to keep everything deep inside, they have no ability to express their own creativity. They may even speak with a lot of pauses, or speak in partial sentences. When others finish their sentences for them, it confirms their inability to formulate and express their own ideas. Because their energy is so internalized, their energy field is fully charged and inflated. But because they have been invaded so often, their energetic boundaries are full of holes, where energy from others easily penetrates. So even though they have built this thick wall of protection around themselves, that wall is actually leaky.

Masochists fear being invaded, and they have a hard time figuring out where others begin and they end. The sixth and third chakras are open, so masochists basically function from their mental and emotional centers. Physically, masochists' bodies will look heavy and compacted, compressed from the top down. They may have a short neck, be short waisted, and have overdeveloped muscles. The throat chakra is blocked, and the head thrusts forward. Their eyes look confused, and their energy stays at a low level even though they may be "boiling" inside. They wind up getting teased a lot, which they hate, as it brings up all their shame and guilt. A classic masochist is Jason Alexander as George Costanza in the comedy series *Seinfeld*. Another is Lena Dunham playing the part of Hannah Horvath in the television series *Girls*.

Masochists carry a lot of pressure on their back and shoulders. Diabetes is a common problem because it's really about too much internal pressure. There is a longing to be free so they can express themselves, so to heal, masochists must allow themselves to feel and to express their emotions, especially the difficult and tender feelings. They have to learn how to be angry with others rather than at themselves, which will release them from being humiliated.

Rigid

The last one, the rigid mind/body type, forms at the latest age, around four to six years old. It's a time when the heart is most open, and these children are rejected by their parents of the opposite sex. It is such a big betrayal that the children learn how to hide it completely. Or the parents tell the children to act more grown up. The children's real self doesn't seem to be appreciated or loved. So the children have to hide their real feelings, which they feel are obviously unacceptable, and simply look and act good, which becomes the rigid defense mechanism.

Rigids hold back their feelings so they won't look foolish; they try to be "perfect" and thus lose touch with their authentic self because they cannot see or admit their emotional needs or weaknesses. Rigids are terrified of being vulnerable, so they don't ever risk doing or saying something that might harm their pride. They focus on their achievements in the world, unconsciously striving for the parental approval and love they didn't receive as a child. But no matter how successful they are in the outer world, they are not satisfied with that. Substance abuse can become a real problem for this mind/body type.

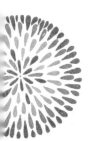

The rigid is the classic type A personality, who is often not sensitive to others' emotions. Career is more important than personal relationships. They look good; they're successful. They seem to be on top of the world. They may go to therapy (although the rigid is the least likely to seek help) but seem to have no problems. Right. When I first admitted I was an alcoholic and went to my first Alcoholics Anonymous meeting, I showed up in $1,700 cowboy boots. Rigids don't realize what they are doing by sporting such a perfect façade. People with the rigid character probably had lifetimes when they kept up an appearance of perfection so they could survive.

Rigids are afraid to have any feelings—those messy emotions!—so everything is perfect—every hair is in place. One way they protect their boundaries and assert their will is to manipulate others through a seductive or aggressive way of speaking. They rarely listen to someone else's perspective, always defending their own. You may notice that their pelvis is tipped back, but in general they've got so much body armor that you can't sense anything wrong. And they have these sparkling, present eyes, with great energy. They are completely separated from whatever pain happened in their past. However, they frequently have problems with love relationships. It's difficult for them to give or receive love, but hey, they look great! A perfect rigid is the character of Alicia Florrick in *The Good Wife* television series, as played by Julianna Margulies. That wardrobe! She's always perfectly put together. Jon Hamm portrays another great rigid as Don Draper in *Mad Men*.

The feeling energy centers in the front of the body are usually closed, while the will centers that run along the back are especially strong. The second chakra might be closed, with the life force pushed into the third chakra. Thus, rigids live mainly through the will and the mind. As healing work is done, the front feeling centers will open more.

The biggest fear for rigids is being embarrassed by their own imperfection. They don't want to be found out. They will do everything correctly, but it won't be authentically who they are. Therefore, they can't experience themselves as they truly are and have trouble connecting to their own spirituality. Rigids tend to be highly competitive and will withdraw if you try getting too close to them.

Their double bind is the thought, *No matter which way I go, it's wrong.* They need to learn to let go of their grip on perfectionism and self-control; they need to feel. When they do, the rigid character inspires others with a daring sense of adventure and great passion for life.

Dealing with Someone Else's Defense Mechanism

Please remember that this system is an explanation about the way someone learned to solve a problem when they were in the womb or as an infant or young child. That response becomes habitual, even when it doesn't serve any longer. Ultimately, the body looks like the defense. All you need to do to get rid of your defenses is become more aware—first of all, to see which of the mind/body types you might be. Remember, you can be all five, or you may have already worked through your defenses and only react that way when seriously triggered. It's not really who you are; it's just a particular way of behaving. Don't criticize or blame yourself in any way for having developed a defense mechanism that worked for you when you needed it.

How should you respond to people who are manifesting their particular defense mechanism? With schizoids, try to help them feel more present, more grounded, more "here." With orals, don't fall for the "help me" pleading look in their eyes; encourage these people to take responsibility and stand on their own feet. For psychopaths, pull your own energy in and down, out of the way of their blast. Masochists are the most difficult to recognize and the hardest to work with, so how you deal with these people will depend on the particular circumstances. With rigids, all you have to do is open your heart—that is what they need the most. Check the resource section in the back of this book for a link to a fun video that shows the various mind/body types in action.

So you've seen the way energy can shape both your body and your behavior. Another way we feel the force of energy is when we come face-to-face with dark energy—whether that darkness is within ourselves or coming at us from others.

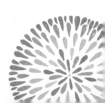

So next, let's turn our attention to dark energy. Remember, you have a slew of spiritual guides at your side, so you'll be able to recognize and prevent or release dark energies so they don't bog you down.

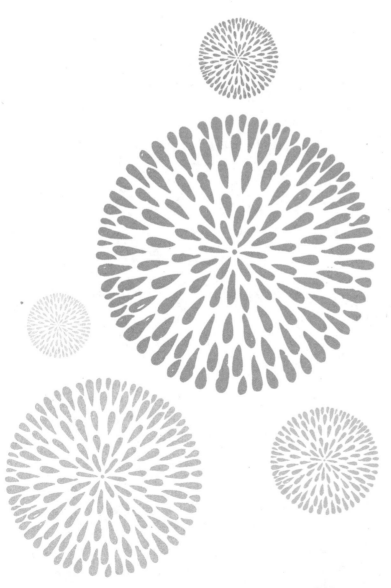

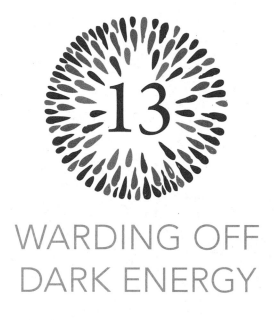

WARDING OFF
DARK ENERGY

We live in a world of duality, where good and evil, light and dark coexist. The truth is, both light and darkness live within us and we are continually confronted with this duality. When you work with energy for the purpose of healing, what are you doing? You are acknowledging and releasing any darkness from within; learning to protect yourself from darkness that comes to you from outside; and infusing yourself, others, and your environment with brighter light.

What is inner darkness? Basically, it is your resistance to knowing the truth about yourself. It is only by admitting your human failings and standing in the light of your inner beauty and wisdom that your energy flows freely. If you see yourself as a failure or no good, this negative image of yourself will cause blockages in your energy flow. By freeing the blockages and releasing the stuck energy, you open up room for the light to come in and banish the darkness.

When the part of you that seeks oneness and the light is more powerful than the part of you that wants to hide from the truth, your dark energy can be transmuted and your life will be brighter. This is the promise of energy healing.

The Dark Side

You are born of the light. Yet even when you were in the womb, you could absorb negative energy. As an infant you could pick up on negativity from the life situations of your parents and caregivers. The less you pay attention to this negativity, the more it grabs hold of you. And then there are your own dark feelings. It's best to recognize your darkness—any jealousies, judgments, insecurities, pettiness, and hatred—so you can release it and begin changing your life.

We all have a dark side. During my own journey, I've had a lot of darkness come to me from the outside. I also created a fair amount of darkness inside myself, especially jealousy and pride, which are classic negative emotions for someone who's insecure. This was a big issue for me, but I learned to tackle these dark emotions by journaling. We can't change what we don't see, so again, the first step is always recognizing what's going on inside you.

How the Darkness Gets In

When you really desire something, darkness will often make you a tempting offer. How far, for example, will you go to get that inheritance, the big promotion, or the top prize? When you resort to lying, cheating, manipulating, or trampling over someone else to get what you want, the darkness wins. And when you give in to using negative means to get what you desire, you become a little darker yourself. But the most damage comes from the lies you tell yourself, especially when you cover them up with your ego and pride.

Each of us has negative feelings, such as jealousy, bitterness, shame, anger, vengeance, or insecurity. If you ignore, hide, or deny these emotions, the darkness can get the upper hand and cause problems for you. So the best way to fend them off is to be conscious of your thoughts and feelings so you can process them and let them go. Being aware of your feelings will help keep the darkness at bay.

You also must maintain your personal power. This includes keeping your mind free of exposure to evil and violence as it comes to you from your environment: television, movies, books, or whatever you're reading or watching online. It's best not to spend time absorbing the darkness of others, even if they are fictional characters. When you allow darkness into your life, it slips into you through the holes and cracks in your energy field. These fissures are there because of the emotions you've left unprocessed and the traumas you've left unresolved. Darkness also creeps into your field when you neglect your body. Abusing alcohol or prescription drugs, eating junk food, and not getting enough sleep or exercise or even sun are open invitations for negative energy to seek you out. Check out chapter 15, "Your Personal Healing Plan," for recommendations to help you out of dark times.

Now let's talk about the specific types of darkness and get some tools for dealing with them.

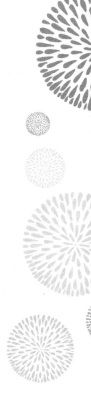

Psychic Attacks

Psychic attacks occur when people aim their shadow side in your direction. It's when your mother-in-law gives you the evil eye or your ex badmouths you years after the divorce. It's when a "frenemy" gives you the cold shoulder because the boss is paying more attention to you than to her. It's when a parent, instead of being proud of your accomplishments, is actually jealous of your success. It's when an abuser or a stalker makes you a target.

When you are under attack, it's hard to stay in balance. You're scared by these people's potential for violence and overwhelmed by their anger or jealousy. And you can't stop thinking about them. It's as if you were tied together in a dance of destruction. Well, you really are tied together. You are corded to each other through strong negative energy.

Cords are streamers of light that connect us to each other, chakra to chakra. For example, if I send out a cord from my heart chakra to you, it will go to your heart chakra. Cords are connected on the fourth level of the universal energy field, beyond our normal three-dimensional space. Even when someone dies, our cords with that person can continue after death.

A cord might be a good cord, as in an exchange of love, or maybe we cord from third chakra to third chakra with mutual respect. A negative cord can be established by any kind of abuse. When I was sexually abused, robbed of my childhood innocence, that created a negative cord from the abuser's second chakra to my second chakra, yet he also corded me in a positive way with love coming from his heart chakra to mine. In confusing situations like this, it is important to strengthen the good cords in order to maintain the relationship. For example, when I started to deal with the effects of the sexual abuse instead of burying the traumas of my painful childhood, I was able to forgive my abuser and strengthen the loving cord between our heart chakras. Cords are willingly shared between sender and receiver. Even though we were negatively corded through the sexual abuse, our connection was basically warm and loving.

The kind of negative energy that people share with one another through cords can be fairly easily remedied by practicing an exercise called the Sweeping Breath, found at the end of this chapter.

In some instances a powerful force that's completely out of your control might be affecting you. I'm referring to vectors of force—streams of dark energy more powerful than cords. Vectors are not consented to by the person receiving them. A vector is like an arrow that's pointed at you; you are vulnerable if you've left a hole in your field from drugs, greed, hate, jealousy—any of the myriad ways that we can mess ourselves up. If someone has targeted you with a vector, some part of your life will feel like it isn't under your control, and most likely it isn't. Vectors, unlike cords, are always negative and are difficult for receivers to release or undo by themselves. It takes a lot of training to be able to remove a vector. If you suspect you are a target of a vector, the Advanced Recapitulation exercise found at the end of this chapter is the perfect antidote.

Again, the best way to keep psychic attacks away is to keep your personal energy field strong by maintaining a healthy body and a positive attitude.

Energy Vampires

Energy vampires use a form of psychic attack that drains you of your energy. They tend to make a big deal out of nothing, thus earning the title of "drama queens." Even minor mishaps become major tragedies. They complain about everything, especially their illnesses. In this way, they attract your attention and steal your positive energy. They may also criticize you so they feel better about themselves. Typically, they blame everyone but themselves for their problems.

After an encounter with an energy vampire, you might feel exhausted, sad, or depressed and sense that your positive energy has been drained, leaving you empty and sluggish. You may try for hours to restore your sense of self by eating, sleeping, or shopping.

Sometimes you're just too nice and feel the need to help these destructive individuals. Energy vampires can lure you in with their shy, soft-spoken, and charmingly seductive ways. Since they are perpetually discharging negative energy, they have a continual need to refill their energy gas tank time and again by siphoning off yours.

It's up to you to avoid energy vampires. The good news is it's easy to do. First of all, spend as little time as possible with them. Learn how to cut off their conversations with something like "Gotta go, my dinner is burning on the stove!" or some other situation that needs your immediate attention. It's also important to stay as calm and detached as possible from their negative energy. Resist the urge to fix their problems or rescue them; just walk away. If you can, it's also best to avoid being in close proximity to them in tight spaces, like elevators, and to avoid any eye contact. Stand up for yourself and protect your boundaries.

Of course, sometimes it's your mother, or sibling, or in-law that is the energy vampire in your life. What can you do then? The first thing is to become aware of what type of energy vampire you are facing. There are five types of energy vampires, which correspond to the five mind/body types we learned about in chapter 12. Each type needs to be approached somewhat differently.

- **The betrayed energy vampire (the psychopathic mind/body type):** The karmic theme of the betrayed type of energy vampire is self-sacrifice and victory in battle. Their experience of being a warrior in past lives taught them there were enemies who may have betrayed or even killed them. They are still trying to win the war; everyone is an enemy, and life is a battleground. Their energy fields are highly charged on the upper half of the body. Their aggression projects their energy outward to anyone in their path. Don't argue with this energy vampire, and don't make eye contact. Lower your voice and make it softer; don't try to change their distorted view of the world. They have to win at any cost; they push you to get you to argue with them so they can prove that they are right and you are wrong.

- **The fear-based energy vampire (the schizoid mind/body type):** The karmic situation of fear-based energy vampires is that these poor souls were tortured to death in past lives because of their metaphysical beliefs or their spiritual practices. The only escape was in leaving the body. They were afraid to incarnate in this lifetime and are too frightened to take up full residence in their physical body. They have a hard time relating to linear time, since they spend so much time in the spiritual realms. When they need to function here on the physical plane, they can become angry and aggressive, and thus turn into an energy vampire. Your best bet handling this type is avoidance.

- **The insecure energy vampire (the oral mind/body type):** These people have been through many lifetimes when there wasn't enough food or love to nurture them. They may have also been abandoned in their present life and are scared of it happening again. They are afraid that everyone else is draining their energy, so they compensate by sucking energy from others. They may speak very softly, so it's hard to hear their long, boring talk. Classically, they are compulsive types who may be overweight or susceptible to all sorts of addictive behavior. They are always trying to prove that they are not worthy of your attention. They come across as helpless and insist you take care of their needs. Don't stand right in front of this vampire, or make eye contact. Don't offer to do anything for them, but do give verbal encouragement. They are living in fear of rejection and abandonment, but don't let your pity for them turn you into their victim.

The passive-aggressive energy vampire (masochistic mind/body type): During their past incarnations, these people were trapped and controlled by others, unable to express themselves. They may have been slaves, prisoners, or those victimized by religions or governments. They want freedom and are angry and resentful that their fear prevents them from claiming it. They withdraw from the world but want others to grant them permission to come into the world. They demand and at the same time resist your input. Others may interfere with their development, complete their sentences, and take them for granted. Their internal world is not clear but rather filled with half-formed fantasies and ideas. They imprison themselves and project loneliness, desperation, and resentment, since they cannot express their anger. They usually want your advice but will reject your suggestions. Resist the urge to give advice to this type.

The robot energy vampire (the rigid mind/body type): During past lifetimes, this type was probably in charge of running things and had to keep up the appearance of being perfect in order to survive. Their outer world is perfect, but their core essence is blocked off as they deny the validity of their inner world. They are usually very successful, have a good reputation and a "perfect" spouse and family, and look like they are in perfect health. Others envy them and come to them with their problems. Robot types never complain. They are perfect, and their world is beautiful, as long as they can maintain the illusion. This type can be best observed from a distance.

The Slimer

The slimer energy villain will hit you with one of the most common types of low-level psychic attack. These are the people who figuratively "slime" you with their negative energy. They can be the guy who cuts you off in traffic or the rude woman in so-called customer service who bites off your head. If your energy field is vulnerable (that is, has a hole in it), you are susceptible and even the briefest online or phone encounter can do it.

So what happens to you when you get slimed? You get thrown off track. You feel lousy and don't know why. Maybe you start coming down with a cold, or your old issues surface and you have a sudden urge to wolf down a bag of chips. A small hole in your energy field is enough to allow negative energy to slip in, and the way it shows up in you depends on the location of that hole. If it's near your heart chakra, you may feel grief as old feelings of betrayal surface. If the hole is in a lower chakra, you might turn to one of your old addictive patterns of behavior. Usually the sliming isn't deliberate and is unconscious on the part of the slimer but that doesn't make it any less invasive.

Exercise: Clearing Bath

There's an easy way to clear slime and any negative energy residue that happens to fall on you. Take a clearing bath: Add one pound of baking soda and one pound of sea salt to comfortably warm bath water. Soak in the tub for twenty minutes. After draining the tub, rinse yourself off in a shower and wash your hair. Afterward you'll feel clean, fresh, and reinvigorated. After a good night's sleep, your energy field will be fully recharged and you'll be ready once again to go out into the world with a smile.

Other highly effective ways to clear slime are to go for an ocean swim (the saltwater will work wonders) or sunbathe for twenty minutes with as much skin showing as possible.

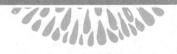

Take Back Your Energy

Negative energy can fall on you anytime and can leave a footprint in your energy field. Maybe someone is jealous of you at work and always tries to tear you down in front of the boss, or maybe you pass someone on the sidewalk who is wrought with negative vibes and some of it brushes off on you. There is a powerful energy technique, called the Sweeping Breath, which will help you get your health and vibrancy back. It is thousands of years old and comes from the ancient Mexican Toltec tradition. The Toltec shamans taught that there are cobweblike filaments (also known as bioplasmic streamers) that project out of what they call the "luminous mass" (the human energy field). These filaments are propelled by emotions. Every situation or exchange of energy where feelings are involved can potentially drain your energy field.

Carlos Castaneda, whose books describe his fictional apprenticeship in Toltec shamanism with Don Juan Matus, a Yaqui "man of knowledge," shared his experience with this technique in the following parable. It goes something like this: When Castaneda met Don Juan in the desert, Don Juan told him to make a list of everyone he had ever known.[1] When he returned to the shaman sometime later, Don Juan had him go to a solitary place and do the Sweeping Breath for every single relationship so he could clear the energy he may have picked up in that relationship and, at the same time, retrieve whatever energy he had left with the other person. It took Castaneda a year. When he came back, Don Juan looked at him and basically said, "You didn't do it correctly," and sent him back to do it again. Chances are that was a symbolic story to show how hard Castaneda worked in order to master this technique and purify himself. And Don Juan sending him back to do it again was the shaman's way of tempering Castaneda's ego-based pride.

Now, think back to the emotional encounters you've had over your lifetime with loved ones, friends, neighbors, coworkers, your boss, or even strangers. You're always exchanging energy with others through these bioplasmic streamers. In the exchange of energy with someone on a psychic attack, you lose your own energy. Add to that the psychic debris you pick up from the other person (especially if you are the sensitive type, as are many healers), and the combination can influence your health and even how quickly you age. Leaving your energy with others, instead of bringing it back into yourself, sets you up for illness, accidents, depression, or financial problems, to name a few. The following exercise will teach you how to get back any energy you left out there with others and return the energy to them that they left in your energy field.

Exercise: Sweeping Breath

This is an easy technique for restoring your energy through the use of your breath. If you're tired, do this exercise another time, as you need to be alert for it to work.

1 **Set your intention.** Sit comfortably, with your shoes off so your feet are touching the ground. Invoke your Higher Self and the spiritual guides whose assistance would be helpful to you (as you learned in chapter 11). Be sure to invoke Don Juan, the master of this technique. Set your intention to retrieve the energy you left "at the scene" with a particular individual as well as to send that person's energy that remains in your field back.

2 **Choose your focus for the Sweeping Breath.** Choose anyone with whom you have interacted, whether someone you love, feel neutral about, or actively dislike; this person may be alive or have passed on.

3 **Visualize the person in front of you.** Close your eyes and visualize the person in front of you in as much detail as possible: clothes, face, and body. Visualize the environment he or she is in—the room, house, car, or out in nature—and try to bring that image into focus. You don't have to see the person's face. Then, set an intention

to retrieve the energy you spent as well as to return the energy left behind with you.

4 **Begin the Sweeping Breath.** Breathe in while turning your head to the left, and then breathe out as you turn your head over to the right. As you keep visualizing the person, he or she will come into sharper focus or you might remember times with the person that you had previously forgotten. By remembering a feeling while breathing in from right to left, your breath picks up the streamers you left behind. Specifically, your in-breath picks up your energy, whereas your out-breath returns his or her energy. Keep focused on that person until there is nothing left to process emotionally with that person. By keeping your focus on that person, you can thoroughly retrieve the filaments and process the stagnant emotions that are depleting your energy. The life-giving qualities of breath give this technique the capacity to cleanse you.

5 **Disconnect.** To stop, do three sweeping motions, turning your head from side to side in the same pattern as before, but this time do it with *no* breath. After you've completed these three sweeping motions, bring your head to rest in the center. This is a crucial step in the process, as it disconnects you from that person's energy.

Know that you are not disconnecting from the person; the process merely retrieves the energy that you left with that person. For example, if you had an argument with your mother, you likely lost a lot of energy during that encounter. You want to retrieve that energy, but you're not going to disconnect from your mother. Doing the Sweeping Breath will help you get some of your energy back and, at the same time, return your mom's energy to her. It's a mutually beneficial situation—clearing a continuous cord of energy you share with that person, not cutting the cord.

Advanced Recapitulation

This is the technique to use for situations when you felt at risk with someone. It could be an abusive parent who beat you, an ex who harasses or stalks you, or a gang that bullied you in high school. Maybe you were the victim of road rage or any kind of psychic attack. Knowing how energy is left behind, even in simple exchanges with others, imagine the energy you lose when you are in real danger or seriously frightened. The intent here is to get your energy back from these people, and at the same time, you will be returning their energy to them. This is not as "friendly" a technique as the gentle Sweeping Breath exercise (see page 154). When you return their violent or dark energy to them, they will have to deal with it. But don't worry about sending something negative back to someone. You're not sending back the event, only the energy that was left in your field. True, it's dark, negative energy, not all fluffy and white. But this is not revenge; it is simply a clearing of energy so you can revitalize yourself. You're not aiming to hurt the other people; you're only seeking to untangle your energetic streamers.

I don't recommend doing this process for someone with whom you currently have a loving relationship, even if in the past that person seriously frightened you. Maybe your mother terrorized you when you were a child but nowadays she's much gentler and you get along great. Don't choose her because it will be too confusing. Try to pick someone you don't see often, if at all. If you ever have to see someone you've done this exercise on again, you will want to be really clear from doing this technique.

The key to this technique is unbending intent. You may already know how to do that through some skill you learned, like winning tennis matches or lawsuits in court. I learned unbending intent by riding my horse. In order to have that giant, 16.3-hand horse follow my directions in a dressage horse show, without the judge being aware of what I was doing, I had to communicate through my intentionality and subtle cues rather than by overtly kicking the horse.

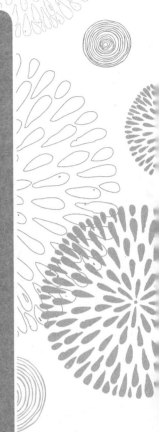

Exercise: Advanced Recapitulation

A key point to remember when practicing this exercise is that you should be awake and alert—never tired—and to keep your vertical power current really firm. Follow the below steps for advanced recapitulation.

1 **Invoke your guides and set your intention.** Sit with your feet flat on the floor or stand with your knees slightly bent (preferably in bare feet). Keep your eyes open. Invoke your Higher Self and the inner spiritual guides you want to assist you (see chapter 11 for how to connect with your guides). Set your intention to retrieve the energy you have sent out to others, bringing those filaments back to yourself, and to send back the energy that is not yours. Focus on your breath and charge your central energy channel (spinal column area) until you feel that you have connected with unbending intent. You gather your unbending intent with a series of powerful breaths. Then you are in alignment and really grounded to the earth. When your intent is firm, nothing can happen except what you intend. There should be no room for any other option. You're gathering your energy, breathing it in, making yourself strong. Think of yourself as a warrior!

2 **Choose a person or situation to recapitulate.** Choose someone who is (or was) very controlling, negative, threatening, or violent to you. The person can be alive or dead. Death is just a change of planes; dead people haven't really gone anywhere. Place your image of this person up in the left-hand corner of the ceiling and leave it there to keep it out of your field. Visualize the person until you have forged a solid connection. Remember to keep him or her away from your direct line of vision and far enough away from your field. Now visualize the bioplasmic streamers, the filaments of light that extend out from your body and

go up toward the person you have placed near the ceiling. Can you tell how many strands there are? Note what the strands look like. Are they thin and fine or thick and cordlike? If you don't see or feel any strands, use your imagination. Make sure to keep your eyes open during this exercise.

3 Extend. Move your physical hand up to the person in the corner of the ceiling. Then, using your intent, reach your "energy hand" past your physical one up toward the person. Do *not* bring the person down into your field. Using your unbending intent, charge your field with your breath, especially in the spine, and start to gather the filaments together in your hand. Use two hands if necessary to get a firm grip on the strands. They will feel a little like vines, or maybe tree branches.

4 Bring the filaments back to you. Keeping a firm grip on the filaments, use a shamanic inhalation—a fierce in-breath through the nose—to start pulling the filaments back to you. It is the breath that pulls them, not your arms and hands. Your hands will know when they should come back to your body. Allow your hands to come down as you breathe the filaments back into your core essence. For women who have been abused, their hands may go to the lower part of their body to return the energy there. Use as many in-breaths as necessary as you grip the strands and pull them back to you in one continuous motion.

5 Clean and expel. As soon as you have completely brought the filaments back to you, immediately shift your focus to the right and shift to a shamanic out-breath—a loud and fierce exhalation through the mouth. With unbending intent, clean off the strands. If there are any strands of energy that are not yours, send them back with fierce out-breaths, using your hands to help you if necessary. This doesn't have to be a continuous motion. Trust your hands to clear your field of any related energies by either sending them back to the person or sending them on to their next evolution. Don't try to see where the energies go; stay focused on blowing them back until you feel clear. It may take two to ten out-breaths. (If you feel dizzy, that could mean you didn't breathe enough or that you hyperventilated. It does not mean you did anything wrong. Just breathe through it.)

6 **Integrate.** Come to rest. Allow the energy from the recovered strands to integrate in your field and in your physical body. You may feel energized with one pass, but it usually takes more than once to clear everything. Check your energy to see if you're up for doing another round. If you are too tired, disconnect and wait for another day or two before attempting another pass.

7 **Disconnect.** Like the Sweeping Breath technique, do three sweeping motions of the head in the same left-to-right pattern but with no breath. Let your head come to rest in the center. This disconnects you from the person and is a crucial step in the process.

These techniques for uncording are really powerful. Continue to use them until you no longer feel any filaments extending from your body. Make sure you drink plenty of pure water and take a clearing bath (see page 152) whenever you work with this process.

Advanced recapitulation may be difficult to learn from the written word. If you are in need of clearing a very challenging person or situation from your field, head to the resource section in the back of this book for a link to a video where these shamanic techniques are taught.

Four Bonus Tips to Keep Psychic Attacks Far Away

Remember, your toxic emotions leave you vulnerable. The more you live in the light, the more you inspire the dark to disappear. Here are four bonus strategies you can use to protect yourself:

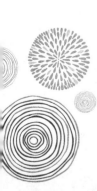

Protect your personal energy and power at all costs. Giving away your power sets you up for psychic attacks, so don't compromise your values and boundaries because you want approval. Be aware of any patterns within yourself that would promote a loss of energy. Always use your own intuition as the ultimate authority for anything regarding your own life.

Keep your energy and emotions clear. Journaling, therapy, meditation, bodywork, and energy healing can keep you free of toxic emotions and dark energy.

Ask your spiritual guides and divine mentors for guidance. A simple daily prayer to your guides and mentors to keep you safe is all you need. I like to use this one: "[Name] and [name], please be by my side today, in every way."

Clear your home of unwanted energy. There are many simple ways to clear your personal space. There are traditional clearing treatments such as smudging, which involves burning sage, sweet grass, cedar, or juniper. If you smudge, open every closet and door, and make sure you circle around every opening; don't forget to smudge the mirrors. I offer another space-clearing exercise in chapter 19 that's even easier than smudging.

In the next chapter, you'll learn about working with the hara line, an entire level deeper than your personal energy field and the source of your purpose in life.

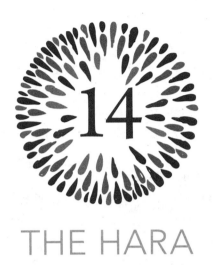

THE HARA

When I was in my early thirties, a shaman I had trained with years earlier was given a message to help me. He checked my energy field by waving a large feather over my body as he hummed. He said, "This is unusual, but it seems you are dying." He was silent for a while and then said, "You have completed the purpose of your present life. If you so desire, you can leave now." After I recovered from the shock of his remark, I chose to stay, as I knew I had more to contribute. The shaman helped me to integrate the new consciousness I was being given, and I began a new lifetime in my same body. Later he asked me if I felt different. He said, "You now have a brand-new hara line!"

What Is the Hara Line?

While your body's energy centers—the seven main chakras—are like a totem pole that runs from the base of the spine to the top of the head, the hara line goes up the spine at a deeper, more profound level.

Your personal energy field actually develops from the hara line, and your physical body develops from your personal energy field. When your hara is aligned, you have accepted your life task, you are living with integrity, and your personal purpose is in sync with your soul's deepest desires. You are well-grounded, with no need to defend yourself or prove that you are right. You respect yourself, others, and the planet.

When your hara line is not in alignment or is distorted in some way, it reflects various problems. Distortions, like splits in the line, reveal inner conflicts. You might feel like you can't cope and want to leave this earthly plane, feel lost or alone or just plain stuck, or feel like you're not able to move forward in a meaningful way. You may have no confidence that you are fulfilling your purpose, and you may even be having a hard time understanding who you really are and why you are here. And you can also lose your ability to utilize healing energy.

Working to align your hara helps to clarify your life's purpose and your task in this lifetime. It stimulates your entire chakra system and energy field. By clearing the hara, repressed energies are released and psychological problems like depression or anxiety can clear up. It's like strengthening your internal tree trunk so you stand taller and straighter and can see where your life is going.

Where Is the Hara Line?

The vertical line of the hara runs right down the center of the energy body, connecting at three main points, the *tan tien*, the *soul seat*, and the *individuation point*, along the way.

- **The tan tien** (pronounced *DAN tien*) is an inch or two below your belly button and is the center of intention and power. It connects you to the core of the earth and then runs upward to the soul seat. The tan tien is a balance point in the body. When you watch people who are really good martial artists, you can see that they are solidly connected with their balance point.

- **The soul seat** is above the heart and over the thymus, just below the throat. This is where your purpose and sacred goals are. Usually the soul seat is no bigger than an inch, but a regular meditator's will be quite expanded. The soul seat connects up to the individuation point.

- **The individuation point** is three to five feet above your head and connects you to Source. If the point is somehow blocked with old, stagnant energy, you might not have any connection to Source or spirituality.

The chakras exist on the fourth dimension, while the thin blue hara line exists on the fifth dimension. What exactly are the dimensions? The third dimension is our ordinary physical reality—the 3-D world our body inhabits. When we are identified with physical matter, we become somewhat dense ourselves and live in the illusion that we are separate from Spirit. The fourth dimension is the astral plane, where the forces of light and darkness, heaven and hell, compete for dominance in your ego. This is where astral travel takes place, and where healers and shamans go to bring back information. When you reach the fifth dimension, where the hara line is, you have entered the plane of light, and now actions are based entirely on love rather than fear. Fear simply does not exist at this level. In near-death experiences, many people find themselves traveling out of their three-dimensional bodies through a long dark tunnel (the fourth dimension) toward the white or golden light (the fifth dimension).

Exercise: Connect with Your Hara Line

Sit, close your eyes, and visualize a line from the individuation point straight down to your soul seat, down to your tan tien, and right into the core of the earth. Now stand up and bend your knees a bit. Point your toes out to protect your knees, and tuck your fingers into your tan tien. Check out the illustration of the hara line on page 162, for the exact location.

Keep your eyes closed. Once again, visualize the hara line, starting at the individuation point high above your head, and mentally bring that thin blue line down through the center of your being, down to your soul seat, then down to your tan tien, and finally straight into the center of the earth.

Open your eyes. Looking down at the floor, imagine the energy of the earth is rising up through your hara line and filling your tan tien. It's important to keep your eyes open when you connect to the earth (and when you are conducting healing energies to someone else) because you need to stay very present when working with the first four chakras if you want to effect change on the physical level. Closed eyes are for sleeping and meditating.

First, see your tan tien as gold in color. As the hot molten energy from the earth rises up your leg and heads into your tan tien, the tan tien turns red. You may feel it heat up to the point that you get physically hot.

Place your right hand at the tan tien and your left hand even lower, pointing down toward the earth. Move your right hand to your upper chest over your soul seat, and bring your left hand up to your tan tien. Raise your right hand above your head and point toward your individuation point. You're connecting your hara line.

Now move your right hand again in front of your soul seat. See how easy this is?

This is a great exercise—short, sweet, and very effective. It pulls the earth energy up into your field. Maybe you don't have time to do yoga or Pilates or T'ai chi, so this is a great quick exercise for charging yourself with energy at any time but especially as you start your day.

Intentionality

The hara line is the axis for your present incarnation and is the expression of your soul's intention for this birth, which includes your life task and your soul's purpose, as well as the ease with which you move through life. Charging the hara lets you live joyfully, in a state of flow. You will be empowered, have a strong inner authority, and know how to maintain healthy boundaries.

Most important, the hara anchors your aspirations, your goals. Your life progresses based on your intention. Everything is possible when you focus on your intention—moving mountains, getting that job you want, stopping addictions, even healing the sick.

I started practicing intentionality when I was a lawyer and would set my intention on winning. No, it wasn't very spiritual, but I learned how to carry through on my intention. You can't float around in an airy-fairy way. It's necessary to have an intention and then manifest it through action on your part.

I further developed my intention when I rode dressage. You don't kick a horse to make him turn—not in dressage. You're largely motionless, using little more than your intention (and your core, I might add) to make the horse turn. And the horse hears your intention. Of course, horses hear better than we do.

If you have a desired goal—let's say you're determined to find your soul mate—and he or she is not showing up, there's a high probability that you're at odds with yourself and your hara line is distorted. One part of you may be saying, "I really want a loving partner," but another deeper part of yourself may be terrified of being hurt (again). There are only two major powers in existence on every level: love and fear. In this case, the fear is stronger.

The Core Star and the Hara

The core star is a point of light that's located in between the solar plexus chakra and the heart chakra. When it connects to the hara line, the core star sends divine light out through your aura into the environment, bringing you into greater balance and harmony within yourself and out in the world.

When you are able to sense the hara line of others, you are on the fifth dimension of the energy field. At this level, you are pure consciousness and can be the witness of their life as it unfolds before you. You sense them beyond time, beyond space, beyond their incarnation in that particular body. As you are flooded with their sacred light, you can feel the qualities of their core star: wisdom, serenity, courage, and above all else, love. It is not grasping or resisting. There, fear is not getting the upper hand. When you are in the place where the hara line and core star meet, there are no problems or obstacles that cannot be overcome with intention.

You can feel the energies of creativity and healing that radiate from their core star as they filter through the hara. You can sense their intentions—and the accompanying feelings, thoughts, and will—coming from the more refined etheric levels down through their energy field level and percolating into their physical body. When both the hara and the chakras are healthy, the individual is open to experiencing dimensions beyond the ordinary plane of existence.

Another way in which you'll reach higher levels of awareness and create change in your energy field is through the simple lifestyle practices that are discussed in the next chapter.

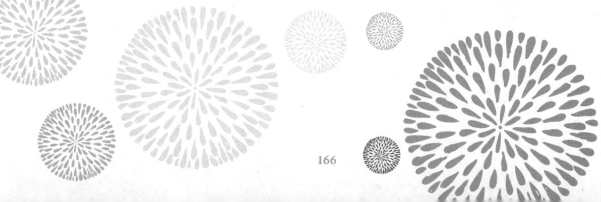

15

YOUR PERSONAL
HEALING PLAN

While some of the concepts in this book may seem complex, like chakras and mind/body types, often simple lifestyle changes are what can make a big difference in your personal energy field. If you are getting enough rest, eating good clean food, not hanging out with negative people who depress you and make you feel bad about yourself, and processing your emotions—these are the things that best protect you and help you to heal. It's so simple that we forget that it's true.

There are some basic practices that will help you to live a balanced and healthy life. You have to be aware of maintaining your body and mind as well as your spirit. Think about the practices listed here and see how you could incorporate them into your self-care routine.

Good Food

There are many nutritional experts with very different ideas of what constitutes a healthy diet. And they all contradict each other. Vegetarian, vegan, Paleo, fat is bad versus fat is good, eggs are bad versus eggs are good, high protein, low calorie, low carb, no carb . . . and on and on and on. The truth is that the foods that work best for you are entirely dependent on your unique mind/body system. We are all different. But there are few basic guidelines that can help point you in a healthier direction:

- Choose food that is "real," not heavily processed. It comes from a tree or is grown in the soil or swims in the water. The most nutritious food will be fresh, local, and in season rather than stored for months or shipped from somewhere else.

- Drink plenty of water, so long as it's pure. You need about a quart a day just to replace the water that your body loses by breathing.

- "Nonfoods" are to be avoided. They have been altered in some way, such as refined sugars, processed foods in boxes or in the frozen food section, foods that have been genetically modified (GMOs), and microwaved food. Microwaving alters the nature of food, and your body doesn't know what to do with it. And we're just starting to find out what GMOs will do to us.

- Chemicals and toxic pesticides are a real problem, so eat organic as much as possible. It is most important to eat organic for any food that contains fat—like meat, poultry, eggs, dairy products, and oils—since toxins are stored in fat. For fruits and vegetables, see the shopper's guide to pesticides in produce put out by the Environmental Working Group (www.ewg.org).[1]

- The body's toxic load is increased through the use of nicotine, alcohol, recreational drugs, and prescription drugs.

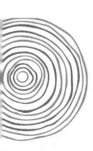

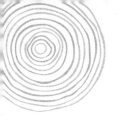

- Eat small meals frequently, especially if you are over thirty years old. Eat protein every four hours, or every two hours if you are under a lot of stress. A handful of nuts or a hard-boiled egg is an easy way to do this. In our modern environment, our endocrine and gastrointestinal systems are heavily stressed (unless you're living in a cave or on a desert island). The best way to support your body is to eat a small amount of clean real food often.

Of course, these basic guidelines are the ideal, but we live in the real world. Choose your foods as best as your lifestyle and budget will allow, and don't get too obsessive about having to eat a certain way. You might start by trying the 80/20 rule: eat well at least 80 percent of the time and not so well the rest of the time. If you are ill, that percentage changes to 90/10.

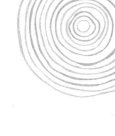

Exercise

Your body's health is dependent on moving it. All the functions in your body—digestion, elimination, blood circulation, and so on—need you to get off the couch and move. Studies have shown that walking briskly for an hour a day can reduce a woman's chance of getting diabetes, breast cancer, and heart disease.[2]

Here are some tips for exercising to support your body:

- Choose a form of exercise that requires focused, conscious movement, such as Qigong, T'ai chi, Pilates, or yoga.

- Get at least part of your exercise outdoors, not just in the gym. Your body and mind want to connect to nature. Walk in the park, do yoga in your backyard, or bicycle around your neighborhood. Your body and spirit will thank you.

- Get at least twenty minutes of exercise a day. You can organize your day to find at least twenty minutes—a walk during your lunch break, climbing the stairs instead of taking the elevator, parking farther away instead of looking for the closest spot near the building.

When you get home at the end of the day, you may be so tired that all you want to do is turn on the television and hit the couch, possibly with a drink and a bowl of chips. Instead, try meditating for a short while and then taking a walk. You'll be amazed at how much better you feel.

Meditation

There are so many benefits to meditation that I'm always surprised that not everyone does it. It puts you in the present moment, relaxes your body and mind, washes away your stress, bolsters your intuitive abilities, and even makes you look and feel younger! Twenty minutes morning and evening are standard. Meditation is covered in depth in chapters 9 and 10, and there's a great meditation practice in the resource section.

Sleep

You probably have no idea about how vital sleep really is. Not getting enough sleep causes major stress, and obesity! If you are sleep deprived even only 5 to 10 percent, it's exceedingly difficult, if not impossible, to lose weight. How much sleep do you need? This also depends on your individual makeup. If you wake to an alarm clock, try going to bed ten minutes earlier each night until you wake up before the alarm rings.

Emotional Clearing

My favorite way to clear dark or toxic emotions is through journaling. By writing whatever you are feeling on a daily basis, you are acknowledging that you *have* those emotions as well as getting them out of your body. No one ever has to see what you've written. Journaling is a totally private and very effective way to get to know yourself better, to be able to see the mental blocks you have, and to release potentially harmful emotions from your field. Another way to release and clear the emotions is through bodywork, such as therapeutic massage or energy healing.

Exercise: Blogging and Vlogging

Journaling is an incredibly transformative practice. It was one of the powerful tools I discovered on my search to know myself better. Initially, I wrote about everything: how I felt about my abusive childhood, my family secrets, how unskilled and inadequate I felt at work, and how jealous I was of all the women out there who were better looking and thinner than I was. Giving expression to my emotions—without judging myself for having those emotions—was a major way in which I became more conscious of what was happening inside me.

Journaling has changed since I started doing it. Back in the day, the tools I used for journaling were a notebook and a pen. Nowadays, you can still do that, but you have other options available too. You can set up a blog on your computer or tablet that can be purely for you, or if you are brave about sharing your journey, it can be made available for others to read. Another powerful way to record your thoughts and feelings is by vlogging—making a video of yourself speaking. Many people are more comfortable talking than writing. You can set up your smart phone or computer to video yourself speaking. You can see the characters played by Jane Fonda and Lily Tomlin using this method in the Netflix show *Grace and Frankie*.

Here are some guidelines to consider for journaling, blogging, and vlogging:

Write it down. For some reason, using your hands to write—whether that's with paper and pen or on the computer—opens your subconscious vault and brings your emotions up to the surface. If, however, you prefer speaking to writing, try vlogging.

Be honest. Don't worry about sounding petty. If you're feeling it, it's your truth. Don't be too critical of yourself or stop yourself from writing something that embarrasses you. Get those feelings out on paper or in video to release the emotions that are stored inside.

Don't stop. Don't pause while you are writing. Don't stop to spell-check or reread whatever you've written. You don't want to break your stream of consciousness. That goes for speaking in your vlog as well.

Find quiet time and space. Blogging requires concentration and a good deal of self-reflection. You don't want to feel rushed or interrupted, so give yourself the space where and when you can find quiet time.

Commit to regular practice. You want to be able to clear old emotional difficulties, but change takes time. The longer you have a steady journaling practice, the more emotionally healthy you will be.

You choose to share. This practice is meant for you, as a way to release your emotions, not in order to share your feelings with others. If you are working with a therapist or have a trusted friend whose opinion and advice you value and who will not judge you for whatever you've written, then of course

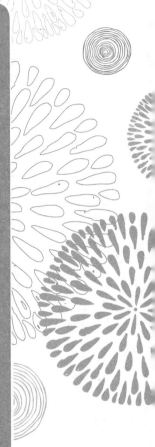

it's all right to share. But it's up to you. Don't let someone trample your boundaries. If you decide to share your blog, you may find yourself holding back from what you really need to say.

Still not sure how to get started? Here is a list of a dozen questions you might answer in your journal:

How is it "your fault" if your parents or children are not happy?

What was your experience with physical, sexual, or emotional abuse as a child? Are shame and guilt still affecting you? Why?

What traumas have you survived? Do you see them as challenges or as opportunities for growth?

How have you struggled with issues related to food, sex, money, drugs or alcohol, or any other addictive behaviors like shopping or gambling?

How did you take care of your own needs while caretaking someone else? Or did you lose yourself in the process?

What sort of a serious physical diagnosis have you had? What is your understanding of the root cause of your illness?

When you are upset emotionally, which area of your body is most affected?

Do you like and appreciate who you are today? If not, why?

What are you most afraid of?

What sort of information has come to you in your dreams? Be sure to write down any big dreams.

Do you feel like some of your problems may stem from past lives? Write what you remember of your past life and its connection to this present life.

How have you forgiven yourself? Others?

Connect with Other People

We live in a disconnected contemporary culture. Even when you see a group of people together, chances are they are each in their own world, staring at their smart phones. Feeling disconnected, alone, lonely, and isolated, is one of the major ways in which people get sick. An important part of self-care is being in touch with others, preferably in person (although social media can also keep you connected to others). We are social creatures; we need to feel that we are part of a family, a community, even a tribe.

Touch

We need physical contact as well as social contact. If you don't have a partner, get a massage on a regular basis, or better yet, hire a professional "snuggler" who will hold you. We need to be touched.

Connect with Nature

Take some time each day to commune with the natural world, even if that means looking out the window at a tree or the clouds in the sky. Take a walk around the block at sunset. Get up early enough to watch the sun rise. Stop for a moment during your busy day to feel the sun shining on your skin or to look, with awareness, at the landscape around you. Really see the flowers or squirrels. Hear the birds. Know where the moon is. In our fast-paced lives, we are really removed from the natural world. If you could just take some time every day to go outside and connect with nature—even if it's stopping at a park on your way to work, leaning up against a tree, smelling a few flowers, petting the dog—you can reconnect with the natural world. We need twenty minutes a day in the sunshine, hopefully as unclothed as you can be without getting arrested, with no sunblock on. The sun is one of the biggest mood modulators. It makes us feel peaceful. That's one reason why we feel so much better after we've been outside. If you live in the northern hemisphere, consider getting a light box to get more rays and vitamin D in the winter months, in addition to the vitamin D supplement you are taking.

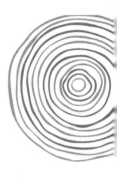

Laugh

Everyone is so serious these days. Lighten up! Laughter is good for the body and soul. It relieves stress and boosts immune functioning. There are those who have laughed themselves back to good health. Try to find something to laugh about every day. At the end of each day, watch an episode of *Seinfeld* or *The Big Bang Theory* or whatever makes you laugh. Listen to some gentle music or read something light and entertaining rather than wallowing in the news and its overdose of violence and politics. Go to bed happy.

Challenge Yourself

So what's on your bucket list? Want to skydive? Learn to play the guitar or speak another language? Visit Machu Picchu? Learn energy healing? We all have things we want to do before we kick the bucket. By setting a goal and striving to reach it—overcoming any obstacles along the way and not giving up if we make a mistake—we develop our will and our personal power. Maybe your challenge is learning to speak your truth or overcoming a particular negative behavior. Whatever you attempt to do, don't get down on yourself if you don't accomplish it. Deep-six the inner critic. It doesn't matter if you screw up. If you don't reach your goal, keep working at it. The real goal is more consciousness, not perfection. You're only trying to improve yourself, not prove yourself to anyone else.

Next we're heading into part III, where you will learn more healing techniques with which you can further help yourself to heal and also help others.

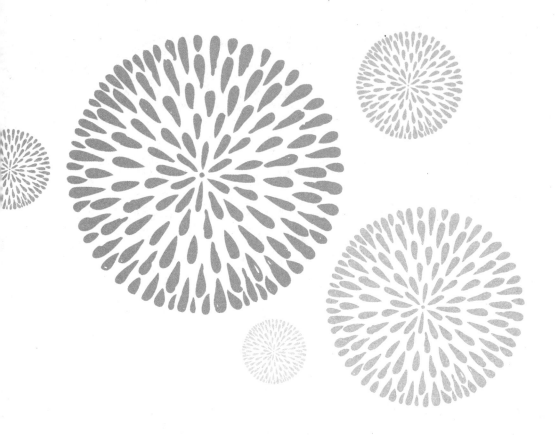

PART III

USING YOUR POWER TO HEAL OTHERS

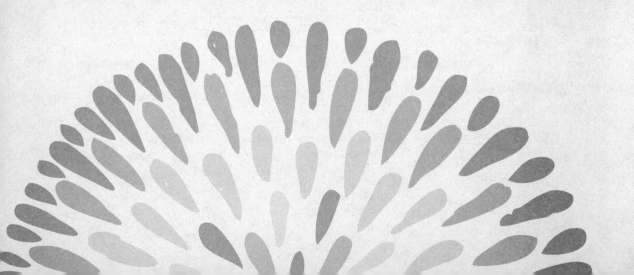

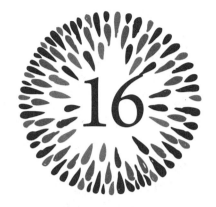

HEALING WITH SOUND

My childhood was dedicated to music. As an adult, I returned to the study of music briefly when I gave myself a term at the Longy School of Music of Bard College in Cambridge, Massachusetts, just to have fun with music. While there, I attended a weekend workshop taught by the conductor of the Paris symphony. He was very gifted. The ten of us attendees sat around in a circle, he would make a sound, and we would answer with a sound; there was no other conversation that weekend. I fell right into this experiential lesson, and I could feel my body changing as it was bathed in this spontaneous creation of sound. After the workshop I walked outside, and suddenly I was hearing full chords and harmonics. Wondering where that music was coming from, I realized it was from the sound of an overhead jet. I had been initiated into a state where music was everywhere, and I remain there today.

Each healer works differently, but for me, the channel I use the most is sound. I actually hear a note or particular chord that tells me what healing channel I'm on. The notes identify which guides are there. I am like a resonating instrument, picking up the sound that's coming in. I listen to a person's body to hear what key she is in. If I hear a particular tone, I know I'm hearing cancer. I can listen still deeper and hear the state of her soul and her deepest longing. I connect to Source and hear which note will help that person, and then I direct and transmit that healing sound to the individual. Sometimes I use my voice to sound out the tone; sometimes I send the tone silently.

Everyone and everything in the universe vibrates at a certain frequency, which we refer to as sound. When you connect with other beings or things that have the same frequency pattern as yours, you are in alignment with them. In other words, you resonate with them. We are happiest when we're around people who have very consistent frequencies that match our own. Our resonance gives us a feeling of calmness and peace. Even better is when we're around people we love and who love us. Love's particular frequency is higher than all other commonly known frequencies. When you are expressing the energy of love through sound, it has the power to heal. The consistent and pure tones of the higher emotions— hope, love, optimism, belief, happiness, joy, freedom, and so on—nurture your nervous system and the beating of your heart.

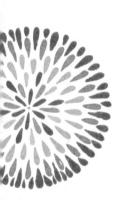

Conversely, when we're around hurtful people who are yelling, screaming, and making loud noises, we want to run because we're responding to their negativity. The sound of fear, for example, is much like a scream. It isn't healthy for your heart function or for your immune or nervous systems. If someone stood near you screaming in fear for a couple of hours, you would likely want to escape the situation. Now imagine subjecting your kidneys to the same frequency as that scream—it's not hard to believe that they might suffer some ill effects after pro-longed exposure, is it? But this is what happens when fear stays inside you for a long period. All the lower emotions—frustration, impatience, doubt, worry, hatred, jealousy, guilt, unworthiness, despair, pessimism, and powerlessness— are distorted sounds that can eventually break down your physical health. Erratic and inconsistent frequencies, such as those from phones, computers, cars, planes, and electricity, can also be distracting and unsettling.

When you are facing a difficult challenge or negative situation, tuning in to your body as if you were tuning in to your favorite radio station will help you reach its healthy frequencies. Raising your vibration is as much about the purity and consistency of your sound frequency as it is about raising your frequency. A consistent frequency means one that doesn't waver. Love, for example, is a pure form of consistent frequency, so when we resonate with the frequency of love, we are bringing ourselves into that vibration, which leaves no room for negativity.

Much like your emotions, your intentions are also based on vibration. The more unwavering the vibration or frequency, the stronger your intention will be. It's incredibly powerful to hold a firm intention to send love to someone who needs healing. However, if your intention isn't firm, you may find it difficult to effect healing.

When your thoughts are aligned with the highest vibrations, they reach the core frequency of love that can be heard throughout the universe. That's why thoughts backed with focused intention are the greatest forces for healing. This premise leads us to the fundamental goal for all energy healers—to reach our core frequency and send out a force of positive thoughts and intentions as often as we can to help heal the world.

Seven Sound Healing Methods to Raise Your Vibration

Sound has the miraculous power to help you reach your core frequency, connecting you to your higher energies and Source, and ultimately helping you to heal. When you are trained as an advanced energy healer, you can change other people's frequency and vibration by working with them to help clear their energy field from any blockages and help raise their consciousness. The key is finding the technique that will help you achieve your healing goals. Here are seven basic sound healing techniques and exercises you can use to tune in to your healing frequency.

1. The Healing Sounds of Toning

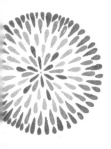

Your own voice is a powerful healing tool for shifting your mental, emotional, and spiritual processes. Toning is the sound of your vibrating breath—a sustained single tone, with no words, no melody or harmony, and no rhythm. It often uses the sound of *Om*, which is said to be the very first vibration that became sound. It represents the union of body, mind, and spirit all in one. The *oh* part of *Om* vibrates at the level of your solar plexus, helping you resolve issues about your identity and purpose while boosting your self-confidence. The *mm* part of *Om* is like humming with your lips closed and is the most powerful sound for bringing you into harmony with Source. Try it now.

Ommmm

Toning helps you breathe more deeply, providing you with more oxygen and opening the flow of energy to keep you healthy and living a long, peaceful life. When you do this toning exercise (or sing or chant), it doesn't just help you—these frequencies go out into the world and lift up your family, friends, coworkers, and all of humanity, which is why toning or chanting is often part of a healing circle (more on those circles at the end of the book).

2. The Healing Sounds of Chanting

Chanting is the rhythmic singing of sounds or words, and it is commonly used as a spiritual practice. Chanting can be highly complex, such as the great responsorial and offertories of Gregorian chant in the Catholic tradition, or it can be as straightforward as *kirtan* from India. There are chants in African, Hawaiian, and Native American cultures as well as Vedic chants, Qur'an readings, Baha'i chants, Buddhist chants, chanting mantras, and psalms or prayers in Christian churches.

Kirtan—which is call-and-response chanting—is part of India's devotional tradition called *bhakti*. The names of God or mantras are chanted to the accompaniment of the harmonium, tablas and other drums, and hand cymbals. Paramahansa Yogananda brought kirtan to the West originally in April 1926,

when three thousand people chanted Guru Nanak's "O God Beautiful" together at Carnegie Hall.[1] Yogananda wrote, "Sound or vibration is the most powerful force in the universe. Music is a divine art, to be used not only for pleasure but also as a path to God-realization. Vibrations resulting from devotional singing lead to attunement with the Cosmic Vibration or the Word."[2]

Chanting may seem a bit out there, but I hope you'll give it a try at least once and see if you experience its healing power. You can find chanting exercises and audios on YouTube and Google Play. There are also many apps available to help support your chanting practice.

3. The Healing Sounds of Chakra Tuning

Consistent sounds, especially pure vowel sounds, relate directly to the unwavering energy of Source. A mantra is a word or a phrase that is repeated frequently. For example, if you kept repeating the seed syllable of *Om*, you would be doing a mantra. When you are repeating a syllable, word, or phrase, you "hear" its sound and sustain that sound silently in your head. The mantra vibrates throughout your body, mind, and emotions. Repeating a mantra can help you cope with post-traumatic stress disorder, help you chill out if you're in a traffic jam, and accompany you on hikes or during your time at the gym. You will recall from chapter 9 on meditation that I give a personal mantra for use in meditation. If you want your own personal mantra, go to: deborahking.com/meditation.

Jonathan Goldman, director of the Sound Healers Association in Boulder, Colorado, says, "The simple chanting of the sound 'om,' or 'aum,' in additional to instilling calmness and relaxation, causes the release of melatonin and nitric oxide. It relaxes blood vessels, releases soothing endorphins, reduces the heart rate and slows breathing."[3]

While mantras work on your whole being, sound healing for the chakras is called chakra tuning. Ancient Egyptian priests used vowel sounds to resonate with chakras, while Aboriginals from Australia and shamans in Native American traditions use toning and repetitive sounds in ceremonies to correct imbalances in the human energy field.[4]

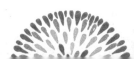

As mentioned in the earlier chapters that explored the chakras, in Vedic teachings each chakra has a particular vibration or fundamental sound, called a bija mantra, that you can repeat to release any blocked energy in that chakra. *Bija* means "seed." So you are literally planting that seed in your consciousness to activate the energy of the chakra. By focusing your attention and intention on the chakra and repeating its sound, you can release any blocked energy. Below are the bija mantra sounds for each of the chakras:

Lam (first chakra)

Vam (second chakra)

Ram (third chakra)

Yam (fourth chakra)

Ham (fifth chakra)

Om (sixth chakra)

Visarga (seventh chakra—this is a breath sound)

Try using these bija mantras if you're having problems with a particular chakra. As you add them to your daily routine, take notice of any changes in your energy flow.

Probably the most popular of the mantras for the heart chakra, the center point of the chakra system, is the well-known Buddhist mantra *Om Ah Hung* (or *Hum*), which is considered to be very healing. The *Om* comes down from the crown chakra with its implication of the infinite and eternal; *Ah* brings in stillness, emptiness, and empowerment; and *Hum* brings the universality of *Om* into your heart.

4. The Healing Sounds of Singing Bowls

There are two main types of singing bowls: Tibetan singing bowls (good ones are made of bell-metal bronze, a combination of copper and tin, while cheap ones are brass and have lots of impurities) and crystal bowls made of quartz crystal. Tibetan bowls are most frequently used to sound a tone at the beginning and end of a meditation session. The sound of these bowls brings a deep sense of relaxation and opens your chakras. Singing bowls were traditionally used in Asia, and the history of making sound with bronze bowls may even go back thousands of years to the Bronze Age.

You produce sound from the bowls by using a mallet moved around the outer side of the bowl's rim, much the same way as when you run a wet finger around the rim of a glass to make it sing. The sides and rim vibrate, creating a sound that has a basic frequency and several harmonic overtones. The sound waves released by both types of singing bowls emit a pure radiant sound that reaches up to the Divine. These pure tones create a vibrational sound field that resonates with and reharmonizes the chakras and the parts of the body associated with those chakras.

Healing through sound combined with the power of crystal possibly goes as far back as the legendary land of Atlantis. Even today crystal singing bowls are sometimes referred to as Atlantean bowls. Crystal magnifies and transmits pure tone. It's one of the reasons quartz crystal is an integral part of telecommunications. Crystal bowls are similar to robust radio transmitters, sending energy out into the atmosphere. The pure tones can activate the brain waves that send you into an advanced state of consciousness and can affect different areas of the brain, releasing hormones and neurochemicals that can lessen pain, overcome addictive tendencies, boost willpower, and pump up creativity.

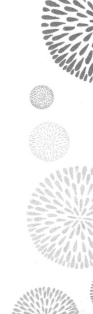

You can find singing bowls on Amazon or in most eclectic bookstores and boutiques. You can also find many YouTube videos that demonstrate how to play these singing bowls.

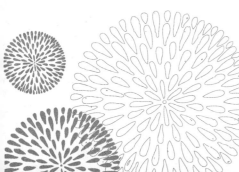

5. The Healing Sounds of Tingsha

Tingsha is a type of cymbal used in Tibetan Buddhist prayers and rituals. In some rituals, the cymbals are used to summon the "hungry ghosts" so they can be "fed" vibrationally. Hungry ghosts are not generic ghosts, like the spirit of your dead Aunt Millie, but ravenous spirit beings with tiny mouths and enormous bellies who represent those with emotional needs that have not been met. Old legends say that hungry ghosts were greedy women in previous lifetimes who never gave away any food. Calling the hungry ghosts and then offering them food, incense, or even a prayer lessens their suffering. In the bodhisattva tradition, enlightenment is only possible after all suffering has been eliminated for all beings.

Shamans use tingsha to clear the environment of any negative or disturbing energies and to bring auric fields into harmony. They are used in meditation and sound healing in much the same way as singing bowls. Generally, tingsha cymbals awaken and initiate healing on all levels and are said to generate an opening in physical, mental, and spiritual reality.

To produce a clear, harmonic sound, suspend each cymbal by its cord, holding it firmly where the string enters the hole on each tingsha. Strike the edges of the tingsha together, usually once, by angling one cymbal at about 90 degrees to the other. Let the tingsha sound until they become silent. You can find tingsha cymbals online, and you can see how to play or listen to their healing sounds on YouTube.

6. The Healing Sounds of Tuning Forks

You may think of the tuning forks that are used to tune a piano, but there other types of tuning forks that can tune your body. All your organs, glands, and cells vibrate at their own specific frequencies, and these frequencies correspond with musical notes. There are twelve keynotes in the human body, and all the parts of your body communicate with each other through sound frequencies. Each organ has its own frequency that will resonate to certain nutrients, minerals, and other sound vibrations it needs to function. For example, the liver produces the note of G, while the colon vibrates to the note of B.[5] If your heart is healthy, it will vibrate at the note of F.[6]

If you think of your body as an orchestra, your various body parts are all musical instruments playing at their own frequency or pitch. If you are healthy, your body will play a harmonious tune. If your body parts are discordant, you can use certain tuning forks to bring your body into alignment. When the right tuning fork is put near the organ or the chakra that is not in harmony, the sound waves will raise the vibration or pitch of that area. Tuning forks clear energetic blockages in the meridians in a similar way to acupuncture.

There are many different types of tuning forks. Classical tuning forks, the ones you'd use to tune your piano, are based on a piano's chromatic scale. Then there are custom-made tuning forks that correspond with the twelve major organs in traditional Chinese medicine, as French musician and acupuncturist Fabien Maman, called the father of vibrational sound healing, discovered in the 1970s.[7] He found that the pitch and timbre of musical notes had the ability to affect a cell's shape, color, and energy. If you can tune in to the "fundamental note" of the cell, your energy field will come into harmony.[8]

Certain tuning forks are tuned to the frequencies and musical intervals of heavenly bodies—the sun, the moon, and the planets. Other tuning forks address specific ailments and illnesses. Some tuning forks make a high-pitched delicate sound that can open you up to the angelic kingdom. Chakra tuning forks are a set of seven forks tuned to the frequencies of the seven chakras. Standard tuning forks are used for toning, releasing energy blockages, and clearing chakras or auras. Weighted tuning forks have a much stronger vibration and stay at their frequency for a longer period of time, so it is easier to feel their vibration. They work well for acupuncture-type treatments and muscle relaxation, and can provide immediate pain relief.

A very simple way of using a tuning fork is to strike it, which sends out strong vibrations through the air, and place it near the part of the body you want to heal or in the area of the chakra to energize it. Tuning forks can help provide a deep relaxation and relief from stress, promote mental clarity and concentration, increase physical energy, integrate the left and right brain, and bring the nervous system into balance.[9]

7. The Healing Sounds of Drumming

One of the oldest methods of sound healing is shamanic drumming, which a shaman can use to facilitate communication between a patient and the spirit world. Drumming is also a shamanic technique for journeying, shape-shifting, and divination. The shaman listens intently to find just the right sound and uses certain repetitive rhythms to summon forth the guiding spirits.

The Greek definition of *rhythm* is "to flow." Various rhythms convey different meanings, while volume and tempo affect the emotional body. The sound and rhythm of the drum creates the bridge that allows you to flow into the world of spirit. Before a ceremony or ritual, the shaman will hold the drumhead over a fire, heating it until the drum is at the pitch the shaman wants to use. The sound waves coming from the drum energize the systems of body, mind, and spirit and make them vibrate in harmony.

Drumming has been shown in studies to have a positive effect on those with Alzheimer's disease, depression, cancer, stress, and Parkinson's disease, as well as those with chronic pain.[10] For example, neurologist Barry Bittman's study on group drumming therapy showed it could increase cancer-killing cells in the body.[11] Psychologist Robin Dunbar at the University of Oxford showed that drumming could release endorphins and decrease pain.[12] Drumming can treat anxiety and stress, sleep issues, fatigue, high blood pressure, chronic pain, emotional disorders, and much more, as well as boost the immune system and deepen self-awareness. Drumming allows us to resonate with the natural rhythms of life.

Of course, other instruments can also be used for sound healing. There's a very old, amusing story about using an instrument to find your perfect note, and it goes like this: In a faraway country, a man played all day on a musical instrument. This instrument had many strings, but he just sat and plucked one string over and over again. His wife said, "Dear, you have this wonderful instrument, yet all you do is play that one string over and over. All your friends have this same instrument, but they play all the strings and create beautiful melodies and songs. Why do you play only that one note?" The man smiled at his dear wife. He said, "Thank you for bringing that to my attention, and here is your answer: the others are busily searching to find their note, but I have already found mine."

Tune In to Sound Health

The wonderful thing about sound is that it not only helps you relax and therefore decreases your stress, but it also can move through any energetic blockages you may have. It can even take care of some physical blockages. I know people who have tried to pass kidney stones, an extremely painful ordeal. When the stone is too large to be passed out of the body, doctors utilize a procedure called lithotripsy that uses sound waves to shatter the stone.

Of course, the ultimate goal of sound healing is to get to a place of oneness, where there is no pain and darkness, only peace and love. When you're in this harmonious frequency, you are in touch with all the frequencies in the universe at the same time. The various techniques I've outlined in this chapter—toning, chanting, chakra tuning, singing bowls, tingsha, tuning forks, and drumming—can help you in sound healing. Although you may find yourself drawn to a particular practice, I encourage you to experiment with each of them, as they have their individual strengths that you may find useful in certain situations.

Next you will learn the fundamental hands-on technique for helping others to heal called chelation.

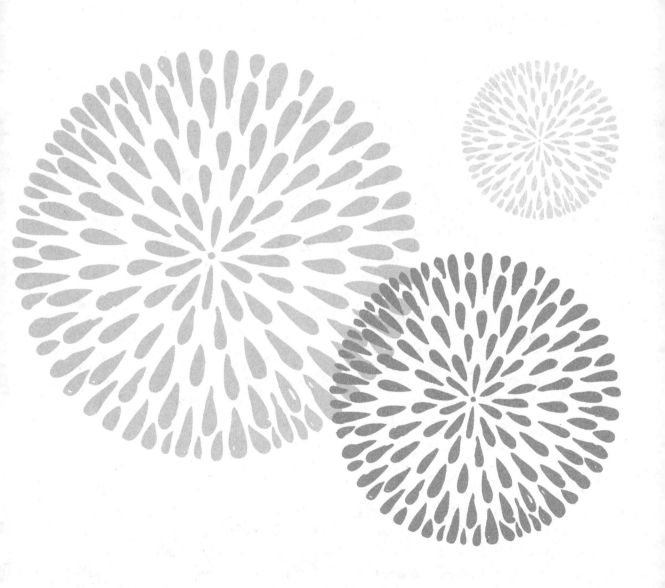

CHELATION AND LIFEFORCE ENERGY HEALING®

So far I have discussed a number of different tools that are available to help you in your personal energy healing. While these tools can also be used to help other people, physical touch is one of the most powerful and direct ways to facilitate the healing of another person. There are many minor chakras in your body, and the chakras located in the palm of your hands are powerful instruments in passing along this energy to those you touch.

Even though the person you are working on is dealing with a present condition, the problem may stem from something that happened many years prior. As you have learned, all physical disorders have an emotional component. Often, the emotional trauma occurred long before any physical symptoms manifested. Your goals as an energy healer are to help clear out the residue of the old traumas, charge and balance your subject's chakras, and aim for energetic balance and harmony. When you do, that person's body can be repaired or stabilized internally on both the physical and emotional levels. However, always remember that this process doesn't replace any treatment or procedures that are medically necessary. In fact, your healing energy will complement standard medical protocols.

Before healing someone through touch, you will want to work for a moment at opening your own chakras as much as possible, so you can not only tune in to the other person and receive the information you'll need to help him, but also access energy from the unified energy field to transmit to him. You also want to establish a solid connection to Source so you are charged and ready to relay energy. The more open and connected you are, the better the session will go.

When you use a hands-on method of healing, your hands are placed on the person. Some areas provide a stronger connection, such as the area of the chakras. If you have developed the ability to sense the chakras of the human energy field, you will know exactly which of your subject's chakras are blocked. If not, you can start by using a pendulum to test the health of her chakras. Remember that the chakras move clockwise when they're healthy and counterclockwise or not at all if they are unbalanced.

I know you've been reviewing the material you've learned so far and you're practicing your favorite healing methods on yourself as well as on your family, close friends, and pets. The only way to become a first-rate healer is to keep doing it. You'll get better and better as you practice.

There are many effective hands-on healing modalities—some are easy to use while others are a little more complex. I'd like to teach you a basic technique that you can practice even in your initial healing sessions. It's called chelation, and it's a great method to use as a beginner energy healer.

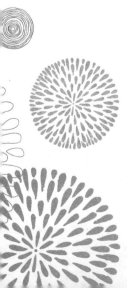

The Healing Power of Chelation

Chelation is a foundational technique that accomplishes three things: it clears, charges, and balances the human energy field. Chelation means "to grab" or "to bind." What you want to do is grab on to the old, unneeded energy that has accumulated in your friend's energy field from unprocessed emotions. In a way, this process is similar to the medical treatment that is also called chelation, which uses drugs (chelating agents) to remove heavy metals from the body. You can also use chelation to help with a depleted energy field, such as might happen to overworked caregivers who never take the time to care for themselves; their field needs to be charged and filled.

There is a certain sequence to follow in chelation to achieve the greatest effectiveness. You actually want to mimic the way energy comes into the human energy field naturally. Your energy originates from the earth, moves up into the soles of your feet, and then heads farther up into the rest of your energy field. When following this natural sequence, your body will take the energy in and send it to where it will be best used. So, in chelation, your starting point will be the feet rather than the area of complaint.

As you work on each area during chelation, you may notice a pattern: a weak energy flow that picks up steam as an area fills, and then a diminishing flow until the energy stops or slows down considerably. When this energy cycle is complete, you know that it's time to move on. Make an effort to get an even flow on both sides of any body part—for example, on both sides of a leg—before moving on to the next area. Likewise, you will want to make sure the left and right sides of the body are balanced in the same way.

However, if you don't sense anything while you are giving a chelation, don't panic. I certainly didn't feel anything when I first started doing chelations. This does not mean you aren't sensitive. It's more likely that you're uncomfortable touching someone else. This fear will pull you out of your body, and you have to be in your body to sense the flow of energy. Your body is your best sensing mechanism, but you have to be fully present in your body to use it. Another reason you may not be feeling much is that your own chakras may not be functioning optimally. The more you transmit energy to others—as in chelation—the more your chakras are cleared, so keep going. At some point, you will sense something, and it will be different each time.

As you charge your client with energy, you may also receive information about her. You may sense something, hear sounds, or see images. If you ask your spiritual guides for help, they may point you to a specific issue. Something may pop into your mind's eye. You might even hear words describing the problem if you are strong on the auditory channel.

During the chelation process, it is possible that your client will enter into a very relaxed state of consciousness or even fall asleep as the energy begins to clear. As you begin chelating the chakras directly, you may find that your client's breathing begins to match up or sync with yours. Once this occurs, you can try to change the pace of her breathing by changing your own. This can be important to do at this stage because the chakras contain emotional material. Your client may want to hold her breath in order *not* to release that material so she doesn't have to experience it. If this happens, encourage your client to breathe to help release her feelings. As she breathes, she may begin to cry. This release of energy will help the chakras to open further and be cleared.

Okay, let's get started.

Prepare for the Chelation

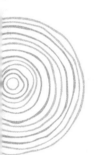

1 **Connect with your guides.** You connected with your guides when you woke up this morning, just before your meditation. Now, briefly reconnect with them, asking them to guide and support your work with your client.

2 **Check in with yourself.** Ask yourself, "Am I okay? Am I standing in a neutral posture, neither in front nor behind the vertical? Am I focused on my client, or am I thinking about my to-do list or worrying about the fight I had last night with my mother?" Clear your mind of all distractions. You want to be in the here and now.

3 **Assess your client's chakras.** Begin your assessment of your client's chakras using your perception alone. Once you have done that, check her chakras with a pendulum, first making sure the client isn't wearing any jewelry in front of her thymus that could interfere with your reading. Using both methods helps you to compare and confirm your findings. Part of your

assessment is to look at the client's eyes. Are they happy or sad? Joy filled or anxious? Tired or rested? The eyes are indeed the windows of the soul, and they can help confirm the state of a client. Have a notebook at hand to jot down your initial assessment.

4 **Gather background information.** When you check your client's chakras, you find may find blockages that you can track to a recent event if you take a moment to chat with your client about her history. For example, you may find that your client has stored a lot of anger and jealousy in her fourth (heart) chakra because a former partner cheated on her.

5 **Get into position.** First, of course, you're going to ask your client for permission to touch her. Then ask her to remove her shoes and have her lie on her back on a surface that makes her at the right height for you, where you're standing comfortably with a straight back and knees only slightly bent; you don't want to have to bend over to reach her. Take a deep breath, focus on your intention to help your client, and activate your healing energy. Stand facing her feet and place your hands on her feet in the shape of a C, so that your thumbs are on the bottom of each foot under the arch and your fingers are holding the top of each foot.

The Chelation

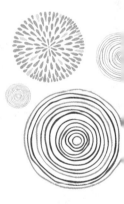

1 **Check in with yourself again.** Once again, focus on yourself briefly and reaffirm that you're clear and present. Ask yourself, "Is my posture still neutral? Are my eyes open? Are my knees slightly bent? Am I really present, or am I thinking about the movie I saw last night?"

2 **Transfer energy to your client's feet.** Focus on your client. Your hands are on her feet, and that connection alone will bring energy into the bottom of her field. Your palm chakras are chelating all the little chakras in her feet. The energy is coming in through the unified field that surrounds all of us,

coming through you and into your client, clearing you on its way to clearing her. Stay grounded. Healing energy comes up through your feet, through your body, and out your hands into your client's field through her feet. As this is happening, depending on your sensitivity, you may be able to feel the energy flowing out of your hands—it may feel warm, tingly, or pulsating. You may be able to feel changes in the energy's flow, such as in the frequency or rhythm of the pulsations or in the direction of the flow. Again, it's perfectly okay if you don't feel a thing; rest assured, the energy moves whether or not you can sense it. Each session feels different—even subsequent sessions with the same client will be different—so have no expectations of what you may sense or feel.

3 **Move the energy up to your client's ankle.** In this next step, if you are right-handed, move around the table to your left, placing your right hand on the bottom of your client's right foot and your left hand on her right ankle. If you are left-handed, you will go to the right side of the table, always keeping your left hand in the lower position. You want to have your dominant hand in the lower position so the energy flows from your stronger hand to your weaker hand. (Going forward, my instructions will be for a right-handed healer—please adjust accordingly if you are left-handed.) As you do this (and anytime you change position during an energy healing), be sure to move only one hand at a time so you can keep one hand on your client's body at all times and avoid breaking your connection.

During the chelation process, you're sending energy that fills you from Mother Earth and from the Divine to your client, and you're allowing it to gently fill her energy field, charging, clearing, and balancing it. Once your client's foot has filled with energy, you may notice that the energy flowing between your hands will diminish. It's then time to repeat the process on the client's opposite foot. You do not need to move your position at the table. Note that you'll be reaching over her body here and thus leaning a little; that's okay.

4 **Move to the lower legs.** To do this, move your right hand to her right ankle and your left hand to her right knee. Allow the energy to charge,

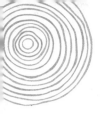

clear, and balance from your right hand up her lower right leg and into your left hand. Again, you may find that at first the energy is weak but grows in strength as the area begins to fill with energy. You may also notice that the energy on one side of the leg is stronger than on the other side. Once this area is filled with energy, do the same on her left leg.

5 **Move to the upper legs.** Continue the process, placing your right hand on your client's knee and your left hand on her hip. Repeat the process with her other leg.

6 **Clear the first chakra.** Leave your hand on her hip and move your lower hand between her knees—this is the position to work on the first chakra.

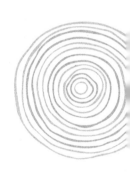

7 **Clear the second chakra.** Take your left hand from the hip and move it to her second chakra, placing it gently just above the pubic bone and beneath the navel. (A quick note: If you are working on a man and you're concerned with where your hand is, just move your hand up slightly so it's over his belt.) Move your right hand to your client's hip. You'll chelate here, first on your client's right side, then on her left.

8 **Clear the third chakra.** Place your dominant hand on the chakra, with your other hand resting lightly on top of it; remain there until you sense the chakra is clear.

9 **Clear the fourth chakra.** Again place your dominant hand on the chakra, but turn your hand vertical rather than horizontal to avoid a female client's breasts, and lightly rest your other hand on top. Remain here until this area feels clear.

10 **Clear the fifth chakra.** Place your dominant hand under the back of the throat, remaining there until clear. Never place your hand over someone's throat, as it will likely make her very uncomfortable.

11 **Clear the sixth and seventh chakras.** To clear the sixth and seventh chakras, move so you're standing above your client's head, placing a hand on each of her shoulders to balance both sides of her field. Slowly move your hands up the sides of her neck to her ears, with three fingers in front of the ears and the thumb and first finger behind, at the temples. This chelates both the sixth and seventh chakras, charging, clearing, and balancing.

Close the Chelation Session

1 **Remove your hands.** To close, very gently and carefully remove your hands from your client's head.

2 **Inflate an energy bubble.** Stepping back a little, put your hands under the table and start inflating a big bubble of energy around your client with your breath. To do this, breathe in and out loudly, more and more quickly, and then give a big exhale. Expand the height of the bubble of energy to reach a few feet above her head. Then under the table, tie the bubble to Mother Earth, with your client securely inside of it.

3 **Return the process to your client.** Step back a few feet from the table and use your intention to return the process to your client. You don't want her to become dependent on you; she's in charge of her own healing while you are only a facilitator. Step all the way back, pushing away with your hands, to signify that you have disconnected from her field.

4 **Rest.** Allow your client to rest on the table for five minutes or so without interruption or disturbances, while you leave the room to wash your hands. After she leaves, take ten minutes for yourself to process and integrate the healing session that just took place as well as to complete your note taking. Let it all sink in. Be sure to express gratitude to all the guides for being there and helping you. Take a few deep breaths and congratulate yourself for a successful session. For a video demonstrating a chelation, see the resources section.

The LifeForce Energy Healing® Technique

One day many years ago, when I was a young student teacher in an energy healing school in the United States, I was called up by the head teacher to take over a chelation she was doing on a client at the front of the room. As I replaced her at the head of the table, I sensed the presence of Jesus, the Master Healer, standing behind me. I'm used to connecting with him, having done so all my life.

He gently moved my arms from the sides of the client's head, where I was chelating her sixth and seventh chakras, and guided me to hold my arms up, bent at the elbow, with my hands on either side of me, at the height of my neck, palms faced up. As I did so, I felt an enormous wave of energy emanating from the center of my chest, the location of the heart chakra. I desperately tried to stay grounded as I was filled with energy from above the twenty-fourth level of the universal energy field. The Master let me know that all I had to do to effect healing on every level, from the physical to the emotional to the spiritual, was to intend it in my heart and allow that energy wave to pass from me to the intended recipient. I was overcome with emotion as I sensed an immediate positive energetic change in the client on the table, a woman who was dying from cancer. Later, I realized that the arm position he had given me was the same position that the Catholic priest adopts during Mass.

I call this technique LifeForce Energy Healing®. It is a great technique to help your family, friends, and clients. I have used it with thousands of people I have worked with over the years at events and workshops and private sessions. It allows you to establish, in a split second, a connection between Source, your energy field, and the field of the person you are assisting; it is extraordinarily fast and powerful.

I have successfully taught students to replicate this technique, and I would like to share it with the whole world. Once you've learned it, you are able, in less than a minute, to attract divine energy, conduct it through your own energy field, and transmit it to the intended recipient. As this divine energy goes through you, the feeling of unconditional love is indescribable. Whatever was meant to happen to your client has now happened. It isn't necessary for the client to desire the intended result, as her Higher Self knows what is best for her. For a brief moment, your energy field has merged with the Divine and with the energy field of your client; for a brief moment, you are in communion. You are left with an overwhelming feeling of gratitude and of being humbled beyond belief.

LifeForce Energy Healing® is different from pranic healing, telepathic healing, and radiatory healing, which I teach in the lower levels of my LifeForce Energy Healing® programs. In pranic healing, you direct your prana, your own personal energy, directly toward your client so your vitality reinforces his. In telepathic healing, you transmit positive concepts and ideas to the other person's subconscious mind to stimulate healing or change the mental attitudes that are blocking him. With radiatory healing, you develop a sympathetic resonance between your personal energy field and that of the person you are working on.

With LifeForce Energy Healing®, you align yourself with the Christ light. This isn't a religious concept. The Christ is the most recent human being who mastered fully opening his chakras and his energy field and merging it with Source. When you merge with that Christ light, you are able to replicate his technique. All you need to do is open your heart chakra 360 degrees (that's the tricky part, for sure!), and merge with him and then with the client. Every fiber of your being is intending, with unbending intent, to merge with this divine light. (Note: You are not intending a certain result for the client, as that would be coming from your personality, which is of a lower value than your client's Higher Self, who knows what's best for her.)

You may have heard the phrase "Where attention goes, energy flows." It's true: energy follows thought, so your strong and positive-focused intention is what powers up this healing technique. The link between you and the Christ light and the person you are healing is inevitable because you are joining your mind and spirit with the force of unconditional love.

It is the energy of Source, coupled with earth energy, coming through you that effects change in your client's energy field and body. He will experience a healing on some level, whether that's psychological, spiritual, emotional, or physical. The exact nature of the healing is up to him and his Higher Self.

While you may be focused mostly on helping to heal your family, friends, and clients, we can't forget our furry friends. The next chapter will show you ways to help relieve the suffering of your pets or simply to make them feel great.

ENERGY HEALING WITH YOUR PETS

love animals with all my heart, and I know many of you share this same deep passion. At any given time, I have had a menagerie of pets at home in all sizes and shapes.

I had a ranch in the Sierra Nevada mountains with an assortment of llamas, horses, a playful pig, Mr. Goat (who traipsed along freely when my horse and I went riding up the steep mountain trails), peacocks, Bessie the cow, plenty of chickens clucking around the barn, and even a pond of fish. These animals were some of my finest teachers; they taught me so much about how to listen to what they had to say below the level of human speech, how to lovingly treat those we live with, and how to heal with touch and, later, with intentionality.

Living with animals of any kind, you come to realize how receptive your pets are to energy. In fact, clearing and balancing your own energy system positively impacts your pets. Although you can't see it with your own eyes, your energy field blends with the energy field of others, including your pets. Your pet is always actively healing you. Especially your cat! That's why animal therapy is so popular around the world and is used in hospitals, children's recovery centers, and care facilities for the elderly. When a friend of mine was in the hospital in Los Angeles, she received a visit from the Portuguese Water Dog that played Bo (the Obamas' dog) on television. He was making the rounds. (Only in LA!)

As an energy healer, I spent many years studying and practicing a variety of methods and techniques specifically for animals. This helped me to be there when any of my own loving animal companions were in pain and in need of my healing hands. I'd like to share a few of these methods so you can be equipped for any animal that might live with you or come through the doors of your new practice as an energy healer. By the way, many of these methods can cross over into the human realm as well.

Using Energy Healing to Communicate with Your Pets

You may not be able to chat out loud with your animals, like in animated movies, but don't underestimate an animal's keen ability to communicate. Animals respond and connect with you in many ways, such as through body language, tone, speech, and appearance. When you listen to your pets, especially in a quiet state, you may receive subtle thoughts, feelings, or images from them. By having a positive, open, and honest state of awareness, and by noting their body language and their expressive faces, it is possible to communicate with them. After all, that's how animals communicate with each other in nature, by sensing intuitively what is happening in their environment. You can trust that they will be honest with you.

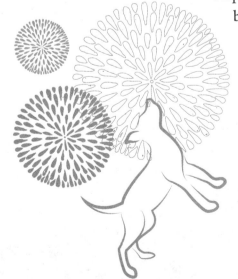

There are four ways you can activate your intuitive power to communicate with your pets:

Sending and receiving feelings. This is called clairsentience (clear sensing), which is a great way of "feeling into" an animal (or a person). I believe this is the easiest sense to develop when communicating with an animal or a person. All you do is intend to tap into the energy centers of your second, third, and fourth chakras. Then tune in to your pet and simply receive the information you need about him. The more you practice this, the more you will be able to sense what your pet is feeling. If an animal is in pain, you may even be able to tell where that pain is and what's causing it. But remember, this is intuition, not medical diagnosis. You still need to consult your vet to verify what's going on and where to head next.

Communicating mind to mind. You can send thoughts mentally and receive them back from your pet in the same manner. This is called clairaudience (clear hearing) because you can hear words and phrases from your pet in your mind. When I heard my horse, Influence, complaining about the hot weather and the way his feet hurt during a ride through the desert, I used this method of communication.

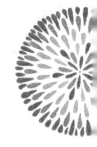

Sending and receiving visual images. When you can send and receive mental pictures and images between you and your pet, this type of communication is called clairvoyance (clear sight). This is a powerful method when searching for a lost animal. You can tune in deep within your energy field and actually "see" the approximate area to which this animal has wandered. You can also use this practice for discovering what happened to your pet in the past. All you have to do is establish a connection and ask this pet to show you images of previous experiences. When using clairvoyance, remember to go beyond the scope of logic as you process the information. Also, keep in mind that sometimes the images you receive are symbolic.

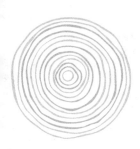

Knowings. As your eighth and higher chakras open, you may find that you begin to receive information that is commonly referred to as "knowings." With this ability, you can immediately receive the information you need to help your pet. However, for now, assume that this isn't the channel you are working on, as it's more likely that you are receiving information from a pet or a person in one of the three ways described above. If you think you're receiving knowings, be suspicious that it's instead coming from your personality; if it is, that information is not coming from a place of trustworthiness and should be ignored. I often find that practitioners in the field of mediumship incorrectly believe they are receiving knowings, when it's actually their personality doing the speaking. But for future reference, when you have been initiated to above the third level, you may well begin to receive knowings. This is the method that I use the most in obtaining information. In this case, the information simply flows into your mind without you even asking for it, and you are given all the information you need to help that pet or person.

Which method you start using with your pets depends on your individual intuitive power. If you're one of the 40 percent who are kinesthetic learners and do best when you're "hands on" and can feel or sense information, then you'll use clairsentience. If you are one of the approximately 40 percent who learn best by seeing, you will most likely lean toward clairvoyance in your communication with your pet. If you are one of the 20 percent who prefer processing information by hearing it, clairaudience will be the way to go. Finally, if you're in that 1 percent group of people who have knowings, you'll get the information that way.

As you work with your pets and other animals, always remember that each of these beautiful creatures wants to be understood in the same way that humans do. What better reason to develop these intuitive healing skills than to help a pet? You don't even have to be home with your pet to know what's going on with her. If you're at work and suddenly intuit your cat or dog isn't feeling well, you can sense into the nature of the problem and send healing thoughts to keep the animal peaceful and comfortable until you get home.

Ways Energy Healing Can Heal Your Pet

Energy healing can help you maintain your pet's wellness, solve your pet's problems and emotional issues, and when the end is near, allow your pet to transition gently and peacefully. There are many ways that you can use energy healing to keep your pet healthy and happy:

- You can build up your pet's immune system.

- You can return your pet to health.

- You can lessen your pet's pain.

- You can speed up your pet's recuperation time.

- You can help your pet recover from a past trauma.

- You can help your pet become more emotionally stable.

- You can eradicate your pet's destructive habits.

- You can make a new pet feel more at home.

- You can reduce your pet's stress.

- You can improve your pet's performance skills.

- You can help your pet to age well.

- You can comfort and aid your pet's transition.

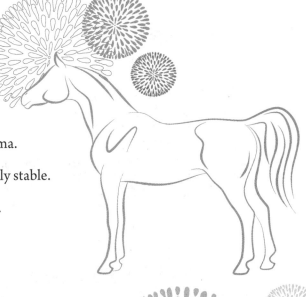

Healing through Touch Can Benefit Pets

The healing power of touch isn't just for people; it also works wonderfully well on pets. This is true even though your pets may have a hard time telling you that they could use some energy healing.

When healing pets through touch, there are a few things to keep in mind. First, certain animals will be very cooperative when you place your hands on them, especially dogs. Cats, on the other hand, are a different matter. Some cats are happy to feel your touch and are fine with the warmth that comes from your hands during healing. Others may be very skittish and refuse to keep still. You can always work remotely in order to avoid being scratched or clawed by any uncooperative animal, or at times when it is hazardous to your health or too difficult for you to be in proximity. If that's the case, you can hold your hand above or in the direction of the animal's body and still be within its energy field. Rest assured, there is no way you can harm a pet with energy healing.

Second, animals' chakras work much the same way as ours do, moving clockwise when they are healthy and counterclockwise when they are not. However, that's where the similarities end. Animals' chakras cycle energy more strongly than ours do. They also have a "key" or brachial chakra, which is an additional chakra that's on each side of the body at the top of the shoulder, through which all other chakras can be accessed. To connect your pet with your healing energy, place your right hand on this chakra and your left on your pet's head, covering the brow and the crown chakras. This will also connect your pet to the universal energy field, making healing much more possible.

Third, size is no object. For example, you may not be able to hold your horse near you on the couch, but you can certainly put your hands on his withers and chest and talk quietly to him. Your horse will relax, which releases endorphins that increase blood flow. This, in turn, carries more nutrients, hormones, and oxygen into the horse's cells—all of which promote healing. And since horses have such huge energy fields, you will also benefit just by being in their company.

If it's a small animal, place both hands on its back, one stacked on top of the other, or put one hand on either side of the animal's body. For a medium to large animal, you might start with one hand at the key chakra near the shoulder and the other hand near the animal's rear. However, there's no need to worry about the exact placement of your hands. You just need to find a comfortable arrangement for both you and your pet.

Healing Pets (and People) through Color Therapy

Here is another healing technique you can use that works best on dogs (people too). Color therapy (sometimes called chromotherapy or light therapy) uses color to affect mood and health. Color is really just light, with different colors having their own individual wavelength and energy. The vibration of the color can affect the energy in your pet's body or in yours. Light comes into our bodies through our eyes but also through skin, so some colors can actually activate hormones and create certain chemical reactions that can help the healing process.

Start by visualizing that the energy you are sending to your dog is a specific color. Keep in mind that dogs can only see a limited number of colors in the blue-violet or yellow-green range, so it is best to use one of these colors in your healing visualizations. The stream of colored light you send out through your hands to your dog can also open up your own energy pathways. For example, if your dog seems hyperactive and isn't sleeping through the night, visualize a cloud of peaceful blue energy surrounding her, or even visualize a bed or leash that's blue in color. And you'll probably sleep better as well.

Colors influence the amount of energy and how it flows in our bodies. As I mentioned in the earlier chapters on the chakras, each chakra is linked to a specific color. Here is a brief rundown of the healing properties of each of these colors as well as the chakra in humans that is most related to that color:

Red is good for bringing warmth and stimulation by energizing the heart and circulation of blood. It also energizes the organs and all the senses. Red is linked with the root chakra and is very effective for loosening and opening up old clogged energy and releasing constrictions.

Orange is linked with the sacral chakra and is warm, cheerful, and frees up the body and mind. It stimulates creative thinking and helps assimilate new ideas. Orange is a stimulating color for the lungs, the respiratory system, and the digestive system, and it gives a boost to the thyroid.

Yellow strengthens the nervous system and the mind while helping to inspire mental awakening. It is energizing for the muscles. Dark yellow is good for shooting nerve pain. Yellow is linked with the solar plexus chakra and can help heal psychic burnout, depression, and melancholy as it carries the cheerful life force of the sun.

Green is Mother Nature's color and can soothe the mind and body. It can be used for almost any condition, since its essence is one of balance and harmony. Its healing properties are linked with the heart chakra, and it has both a soothing and energizing effect on the heart. Green is also excellent for hormonal imbalances.

Cobalt blue has cooling, astringent healing properties. It brings down inflammation, calms strong emotions, and can be used for any problems with communication or the throat. It is linked with the throat (fifth) chakra.

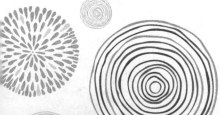

Violet is linked with the third eye and is highly beneficial for mental problems. It purifies the bloodstream and helps with difficulties of the ears and eyes. Leonardo da Vinci once wrote that if you meditate under a gentle violet ray, like sitting in the light streaming from a stained glass window, the power of your meditation and prayer will increase tenfold.[1]

White is the color of transmutation and transformation. Linked to the crown chakra, white brings spiritual renewal and deep insight. It can lesson sensitivity to pain and help in detoxification. White, of course, is the perfect color, for it combines all other colors in completely balanced harmony. White light raises consciousness, and directing white light to the part of the body that needs help is one of the quickest ways to effect healing. If you can't decide which color to use, you can always use white, since its frequency comprises all the other colors of the rainbow. As an energy healing rule of thumb, visualize your energy in white when opening and closing any healing session, no matter which other colors you use in between.

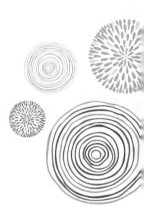

If you know what your pet's problem area is, you can work with the appropriate color in a variety of ways: you could use an orange towel to dry off your dog after a cold, wet walk; get a pet bed, leash, or collar in the color needed; or use colored light bulbs or a colored filter over a lamp and shine the light on your pet.

Working with light, in all its different colors, can fill you with healing energy and lead you to a tremendous experience of transformation that can alter your life!

Healing Your Pets through Sound Healing

Animals respond wonderfully to sound healing, which we discussed in chapter 16, because they hear more octaves and tones than humans do. They are also very sensitive to calm and soothing music, which can reduce their pain and anxiety. I'd suggest using Tibetan singing bowls, since they generate tones that

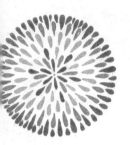

particularly resonate with animals. The sound emanating from these singing bowls can deeply relax your pets and help balance their chakras. Some pure sounds can also lessen their pain and increase their energy.

Healing Your Pets with the Power of Affirmations

Affirmations are a wonderful tool in your healing kit. Affirmations are a great way to send powerful positive intentions and thoughts to your pets, such as the following:

You are healthier than you've ever been before.

You are appreciated and loved.

I listen deeply to you and hear your needs and wishes.

You are wide open and very receptive to healing energy.

You are relaxed and anxiety-free.

You are safe.

I love you more and more each day.

Raising Energetically Healthy Pets

You share and exchange energy with your pets, so let's keep that energy healthy, happy, and balanced all around. Here are a few more tips on how to care for your pets and keep all of you feeling good:

Feed your pets natural foods. Animals are as sensitive as humans to unnatural additives, colorings, and preservatives. They may be allergic to some of these harmful chemicals used in many brands of commercial pet food, which could lead to behavior problems, excess weight gain, or dental issues. Holistic vets recommend natural diets, like raw foods, for cats and dogs.

Give your pets pure water. If your pets are not drinking enough pure water, it will affect both their health and their energy field. The smell or taste of tap water may not be appealing to them, so try filtered water or still (non-bubbly) mineral water. Beef broth or other meat broths, served cool, are another way to get your pets to drink more.

Let the sun shine on your pets. Animals need sunshine for health as much as we do. Pets need to go outside for at least an hour a day to prevent depression, lethargy, and illness. Full-spectrum lighting has been used to prolong the lives of hamsters with heart disease. Keep both you and your pet healthy by going outdoors in the sunshine for a walk. If you have indoor pets, make sure they can access a place in the sun by a window.

Be a friend to your pets. Just like us, pets need companionship. Animals get lonely, so they love being around people and sometimes even other pets. I actually got a mini—a small horse—to keep my big horse, Influence, company when his pet goat passed on. Some pets, such as rabbits, gerbils, birds, fish, guinea pigs, and even rats, do best in same-sex pairs. Hamsters, on the other hand, are happiest by themselves in their own little world. Some pets, like llamas, will really become despondent if they don't have the companionship of another llama; you'll want to be informed about its needs before you choose an exotic pet.

Give your pets space. All pets need lots of room to move around easily. We cannot imprison our pets in cages, pens, or runs that are too small. However, some dogs feel safest in a "den," like a crate or kennel for sleeping. Listen to your animals' needs and act accordingly.

How Helping Your Pets Can Help You

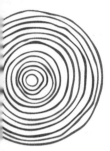

When you aim energy healing in the direction of your loving pets, much of that healing mojo will come right back to you. All you have to do is show a little love for an animal; merely petting it on the head will automatically produce a hormone in you that activates your nurturing abilities. And this is just the tip of the iceberg—innumerable studies are now being conducted on the powerful connection between owners and their pets. You'd be amazed to learn how much making a conscious effort to heal and connect with your pets will benefit you in return.

The Healing Power of Cats

Unlike canines, the felines of the world can be difficult to read during an energy healing. Yet cats play a vital role in the life of an energy healer as they have quite a bit of power, and can teach you many lessons.

Cats are the foremost mystical members of the pet family. In ancient Egypt and China, cats were revered as goddesses. It was believed that they were able to sense a person's energy field and keep those around them in balance. In Japan, cats are also known for their extraordinary power. Whenever a vessel sets out to sea, a cat accompanies the crew to ward off bad spirits as well as to attract wealth. Even today, the Maneki Neko—a three-colored cat—is a welcome crew member on Japanese ships.

In Buddhist teachings, it is said that Buddha loved cats and that these felines would often serve as a temporary refuge for the souls of very spiritual people. Buddhists continue to have a high regard for cats and revere these sacred animals, both in their lives and in their prayers.

Ancient civilizations also believed cats had occult abilities, such as being able to watch a ghost as intently as they watch a flesh-and-bone human being. If they saw a benign being, the cats would be restless but not overly upset. However, if the ghostly visitor intended to do harm, the cats would hiss and spit at the intruder. It is still believed that mystical cats guard you from unwanted spirits while you sleep, which is why they want to sleep on your bed. Cat owners feel a sense of peace when their cat is happily curled up next to them or on their lap. It's a deeper sense of tranquility than the exuberant welcome home you receive from your dog.

As an energy healer, you can still use many healing techniques on your cats, including touch and sound healing. But you'll probably find that cats work much better on the flip side of the process . . . as the healer themselves! All cats have the ability to release any negative energy you've accumulated in your body during the day, and they can purr away any negativity while you sleep. While they sleep, that negativity is released from the cat's body. If you're highly stressed, your cat may not be able to release the negative energy all at once, so it is stored until she has enough time to process it.

Welcome Animals to Your Healing Team

As an energy healer, you definitely want your pets on your personal healing team, since they use their acute natural powers to enhance your health. Whenever I am with my much-loved Influence, whether I am grooming and petting him or just in his presence, that huge horse always grounds me. Even when I'm not around him, I am still able to mentally connect my energy field to his. I know many people who have this type of relationship with their animals—dogs or cats, or even birds or fish.

In addition, pets are great to practice on when you're learning how to heal people. Many healers, including myself, will affirm that they did some of their healing training with the willing help of their animal companions. With all that our pets do to help keep us healthy and psychologically sound, it's important to remember to return the favor whenever we can.

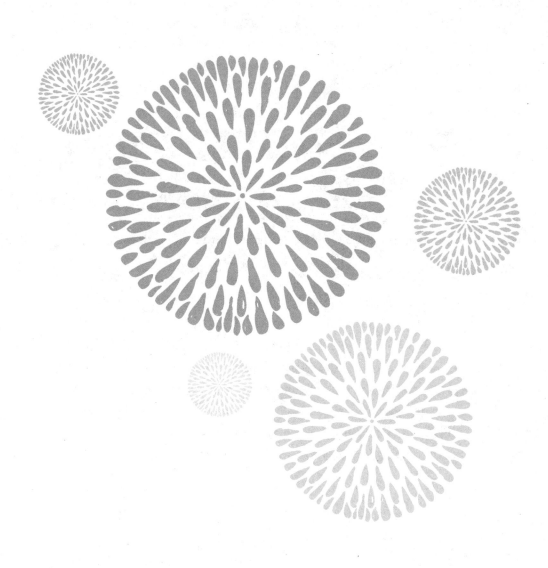

SHARE YOUR GIFT OF ENERGY HEALING

Congratulations! I am very proud of you for sticking with me, embracing these teachings, and getting to the last chapter in this book. Most important, I applaud you for recognizing the healing power within you and wanting to share it with the world. I'd like you to stand up right now and walk over to a mirror. Take a close look at that talented, magnificent, and confident person smiling back at you. Look deeply into your eyes and say, "I have the power to heal." Say it again with all your heart and all your chakras bursting forth with passionate energy, and then, "I can help heal the world."

Working in the healing arts combines service on the physical, emotional, psychological, and spiritual levels. Even if your work with energy healing is focused on healing *you* and not on becoming a professional energy healer, that also serves the greater good. Energy healing is an integral part of your personal spiritual path, and as you become more conscious, that in itself helps to awaken humanity.

As you delve deeper into the realm of energy work, you'll come to understand that we're all interconnected. When you realize this concept of unity, you'll understand that it's really important to help others and care for all creation. When you know that the divine Source is within each person, you will be drawn to help anyone who is suffering and in need of help.

Doing healing work is selfless service. The selfless part means you are doing your work in order to relieve suffering, not because of what you might gain personally. It's like feeding the homeless because you believe everyone deserves to eat, not because it makes you look like a humanitarian. The Bhagavad Gita (5:12) says, "This man of harmony surrenders the reward of his work and thus attains final peace: the man of disharmony, urged by desire, is attached to his reward and remains in bondage."[1]

In selfless service, you begin to understand people—their challenges, life circumstances, hopes, and dreams. Each one of us has either deliberately or inadvertently hurt others in the course of our life. Can you say that you've never cheated, stolen, lied, or done something immoral? Of course not. Being of service to others is a great way to make amends. His Holiness the Dalai Lama, the well-loved spiritual leader of Tibetan Buddhists, has said many times that his religion is "kindness" and that the purpose of life is to help others. Service also gives rise to humility—knowing in your heart that you're not more spiritual, higher, or better in any way than those you serve. Authentic energy healers seek to make the world more harmonious and to broaden their capacity to love and serve, not bolster their egos.

If you want to be of service, you first have to learn to take good care of yourself. You can't share energy you don't have. This means you can't stop using energy healing tools—meditation, clearing your chakras, connecting with your spiritual guides—for your own healing because you're too busy helping others. Caretakers are frequently in this position and eventually burn out. Even if you start with the best of intentions, you may wind up feeling angry and resentful toward the people you are caring for. Remember, taking care of yourself is not the same as being selfish, and you should never feel guilty about maintaining your own health and happiness.

Energy healing is a cocreative process between you, the person who is being healed, and Source. As an energy healer, your service to humanity is to act as the conduit for tapping into the universal energy field and directing that energy toward the person you are helping to heal.

Preparing for a Healing Session

When you believe you're ready to start treating friends and family, the first thing you must do is find an appropriate setting—a space that promotes healing. Make sure the ambience is quiet, private, and relaxing. You can start at home, dedicating a room as your healing space. You can decorate this room in soothing tones and add harmonious elements, such as a small Buddha or another representation of the Divine. Make it a place where your clients will feel safe and comfortable.

Then you'll want to make sure your space is clear of any negative energies. The following is one way to clear your space safely using a visualization technique.

Exercise: Clearing Your Space

Stand comfortably in the space you want to clear. Take some slow, deep breaths to center yourself.

Now picture a white tablecloth or sheet beneath your feet. It's as big as the whole space you are in. Use your intention to visualize that sea of white cloth beneath you.

Using your energy and with focused concentration, start to raise the white sheet off the floor. It will go right through you because it's energy. What you're actually doing is using your intention to raise all the dark energy in your space up, up, and away. The white sheet will take away anything that is depressing, negative, sad, or anxious within your space and within you.

Using your breath, keep raising the white sheet. It's like a big parachute, ultimately rising above you. Watch it as it floats up. Push it above the ceiling and up over the roof. And away it goes!

When someone comes to you for a session, make sure your electronics (and theirs) are turned off. You don't want ringing phones, text or email alerts, or stray noises from a television or computer interrupting the flow of healing energy. And even though you may be convinced that your dog or cat is also a great healer, you must keep pets out of the space. Animals have an instinctive inclination to tune in to the energy around them and take it for themselves.

Conducting the Healing Session

When someone asks you for energy healing, take a few minutes when he first arrives to talk to him about any problems he may wish to address. Use your intuition to determine the state of his chakras, and then your pendulum to check the accuracy of your intuition. For example, if your client is complaining of stomach pains, and he has been examined medically and there is no obvious physical cause of the pain, you can check his chakras to see if there is something blocking the flow of energy in or around his third chakra. Or if someone shows up lamenting her betrayal by her best friend at work, you'll be conscious of the possibility of problems in the third and fourth chakras.

When you've completed your intake and your review of the person's energy field, you're ready to get started. You'll want to have an open mind about what will happen during the session. Perhaps you start with a chelation but are guided midway to begin toning. Or maybe you begin seated, in a coaching format, and then are guided to lead your client to do a healing. Just about anything can and will happen during a session, and each one will be different even if it's the same client.

Remember that you can use energy healing in a very collaborative way with traditional medical therapies. Always be respectful of the valuable benefits that other healthcare professionals can provide, referring your clients to them when appropriate. It's important to know your limitations and never diagnose or treat medical conditions. The people you work with are your *clients*, not your *patients*. You can talk about the goals of energy healing as the clearing, balancing, and charging (energizing) of your client's field, never about curing anything. You assess (not diagnose) your client's chakras and energy field and *suggest* (not prescribe) possible solutions.

Keep in mind that your client's Higher Self knows best and knows way more than you. Your personality needs to take a backseat throughout; this is actually the hardest step for a burgeoning energy healer to learn. The moment you think you know what's best for your client and feel the urge to tell him so (in no uncertain terms!) is the moment you have slipped out of healership and into ego. The more you feel inclined to share what you are sensing about your client with him, the more you are in ego; over-sharing is the sign of a novice energy healer. An experienced energy healer tends to work in silence, feeling no need to be validated for her insights and gifts. That experienced practitioner knows she can do the work and feels no need for approval.

You will want your clients to have a clear understanding of your policies and procedures. Let your clients adjust how the session is going or end the session at any time. Never force something on clients that they don't want. Don't engage them in conversation at the end; rather, let them integrate in silence. Don't assume they want to book another session; let them make that decision after they return home. Remember, the session is about the client. You do this work because you *can*, not because you need approval.

Be Ethical

Because energy healing is a business with no outside organization to set industry standards, it is of vital importance to be ethical. You are impacting another person's life, so you have to be very aware that whatever you do, you are doing it for the person's highest good.

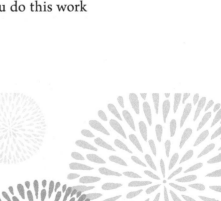

Part of being ethical involves telling the truth and never intentionally misleading your clients about what they can expect from you or the healing process. If, by chance, it turns out that you are not compatible with a client, suggest someone more appropriate. For example, you may choose to refer groups in corporate environments to another practitioner because your training and skills are more appropriate for working mainly with individuals on personal matters.

Being ethical also means keeping private information secure. Since you will be hearing personal information from your clients, you are responsible to keep absolutely everything that is said completely confidential. This includes protecting your session records so no one but you can access them. Protecting confidential information is a vital part of the ethics of being an energy healer.

There are three main principles that will ensure you are being ethical with your family, friends, and clients:

- **Permission:** Start every session by asking, "How may I help you?" It's a reminder that you and your client will be working together to bring about any change. It's very important to have your client's permission before proceeding with a session, and this simple question gives you that permission.

- **Positive outcome:** Always approach each session with an open heart and open spirit. Remind your client about the positive outcome she can achieve. If you feel dark energy in the person, don't mention it. Instead, handle the situation in silence because you never want to make your client feel fearful. More important, there's a strong chance that you could be wrong; novice energy healers are inclined to think they are sensing dark energy when it's really they who are triggered by the session, and it's their own darkness they are sensing.

- **Separate your fields:** At the end of the session, always separate your energy field from the client's—in your mind and energetically. Acknowledge that your client is able to care for himself.

Listen to Your Gut Feelings

It's rare that any problems will get in the way of your new energy healing work, but you want to be prepared for the unexpected. What do you do if there's a healing session that doesn't feel right to you, or if there's a request for a session that takes you out of your comfort zone? When you're faced with any sensitive or difficult situations, always center and quiet yourself, look within, and listen to your inner wisdom.

For example, imagine one of your clients sends a friend or relative to see you. When the person arrives for her first session, she tells you about her struggle with her inner demons and the medications she has taken for anxiety and depression. Suddenly she says something that makes you realize she is one of your children's teachers. What do you do? Your values will help you determine the right course of action to take. Are you worried that this teacher may have a negative influence on your child? Do you pull your child from her class? Or do you admit your personal connection right away and recommend she see someone else? There is often no simple answer when presented with an ethical dilemma. All you can do is listen within to see which option feels right to you.

As an energy healer, you want to be known for your skill and integrity, the same qualities that will ultimately lead you in the right direction. Your clients will notice that you walk your talk. Examine your values; act on the best of them, and your practice and life will lead you to mastery.

Tips for When You're Ready to Take on Paying Clients

After you have practiced on yourself and your friends and family and pets for a prolonged period of time and feel comfortable with the various aspects of energy healing, you may decide you are ready to take on paying clients. Once you make this decision, there are a few things that you need to keep in mind.

Charging fees can be a difficult area for energy healers. To reduce the chances of confusion or conflicting expectations, it's important for both you and the individuals you are working with to be up front about your fees and billing arrangements. It may feel slightly uncomfortable, but charge what you think your services are worth, being fair to your clients as well as yourself. You can also research the field and compare your rates to others in your area. Of course, when you're first starting out, you may not want to be the most expensive energy healer in your area. Stay within your ethical boundaries and you will be known as a reputable energy healer.

It's best to handle the money part separate from the session so as not to engage your clients in thought when they are integrating; consider using one of the many web-based solutions that allow your clients to both make their appointment and pay for the session online.

You will also need to look into licensing requirements in your area. You don't need any sort of license to use your healing abilities on your family and friends, as you are not charging them for sessions, but most jurisdictions require a license if there is to be any touching or an exchange of money. You will want to consider certification, whether you are required to be licensed or not. Certification from a recognized school (see the resource section at the end of this book to learn about my own school) demonstrates a professional level of competency and legitimacy, and lets clients know that you are educated in the art of healing. Also, as a certified energy healer, you will attract more clients and increase your earnings.

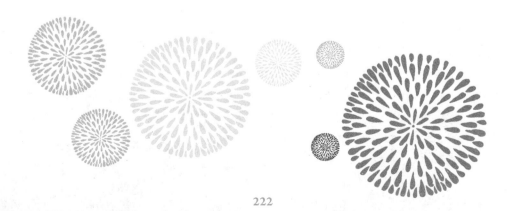

CONCLUSION
HEALING CIRCLES

Learning, experiencing, and embodying what it means to work with energy healing on a personal or professional level is just the tip of the iceberg. Ultimately, what you have learned and experienced about energy healing in the course of this book can be used to help heal the world. There is immense power when a group of people, however small, gets together with the same positive intention to heal in their minds and hearts.

In my first book, *Truth Heals*, I tell a story that, to this very day, continues to shape the direction of my work as a healer:

> I once heard a story about an aboriginal tribe that conducts a healing ceremony whenever anyone in the village is sick. The person with the high fever or the stomach ailment or the depression or the congested lungs sits in the center of a circle of all the villagers. The sick person is invited to speak the things *that have been left unsaid* by directly addressing those he felt harmed by or whom he had harmed with words or actions. What has been weighing on his heart that has never been shared? What dreams have been suppressed? The person speaks his truth. The villagers listen and acknowledge what has been said; they sit in the circle with the person who has been sick until that person is well. The tribe knows what we as a culture have forgotten: *truth heals.*[1]

I've experienced this same phenomenon in the workshops I hold and in the healing circles that are part of my LifeForce Energy Healing® program. If you've ever attended one of my in-person events or online video workshops, you already know what I mean. You've witnessed the physical, emotional, and spiritual transformation that happens in that setting. You've watched participants release decades of buried shame, guilt, and regret. You've seen faces in anguish become suddenly serene as the vision of a beautiful, joy-filled, and abundant future unfolds before them. I bet you've experienced this kind of transformation on occasion yourself: perhaps in a church, temple, or ashram or at a 12-step meeting where the stated intention was to heal.

I want you to know that you can harness that same power right now, whenever and wherever you need by forming your very own healing circle.

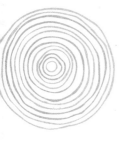

Healing Circles

A healing circle is a group that prays and meditates together to give or receive healing on any level—psychological, physical, emotional, or spiritual. For instance, Buddhist healing circles may chant the Medicine Buddha mantra for those who need healing. The energy generated by a healing circle is transformational. The vibrations sent out by a group praying or meditating or chanting together are more powerful than those sent out by an individual. As the Master Healer said, "Where two or three gather in my name, there I am among them" (Matthew 18:20).

Numerous cultures throughout the world have used healing circles. In the language of the Lakota tribe, healing circles are called *hocokah*, which means "sacred circle" and is also the word for "altar." The hocokah is a circle of people who sit together to pray and perform ceremonies, and they are deeply committed to helping each other's healing. These kinds of circles have proven helpful, especially in recovery from alcoholism. In Native American beliefs, the circle is often called the medicine wheel—the way of harmonizing with the movement of the circle and living, breathing, and moving in balance with the environment.

My initial adult experience of a healing circle took place when I first went to Alcoholics Anonymous. At the end of the meeting, everyone stood in a circle and joined hands while reciting the Serenity Prayer: "God grant us the serenity to accept the things we cannot change; courage to change the things we can; and wisdom to know the difference."[2] It was truly powerful!

Every healing circle you initiate provides the essentials for massive shifts in consciousness and positive change in the world. You have everything you need to make a difference, but you have to believe in your potential for creating positive change.

Worldwide Healing Day

Mahatma Gandhi is reputed to have said, "Be the change you wish to see in the world." However, that was really an encapsulation of what he actually said, which was:

> We but mirror the world. All the tendencies present in the outer world are to be found in the world of our body. If we could change ourselves, the tendencies in the world would also change . . . This is the divine mystery supreme. A wonderful thing it is and the source of our happiness.[3]

Here's your chance to be that change he spoke of. Join me in celebrating Worldwide Healing Day. I was inspired by my publisher to create such a day and to make it an annual tradition. The first one is scheduled to coincide with the publication of this book. We will join together in a meditation to heal the world. Imagine the healing power we can generate together. Let's awaken ourselves along with our local and global communities to the limitless power of healing!

You are ready to begin your magical new journey as an energy healer. The time is now. The only place you can create positive change is in the present. The past is over with and cannot be changed. The future has yet to happen, and what you do in the present will alter that future. So the only time you can work on yourself or others is in the *now*. In *Gone with the Wind*, Scarlett O'Hara could get away with thinking about it tomorrow. As she says in the very last line of the movie, "After all, tomorrow is another day."[4] But we can't afford to wait until tomorrow, not if

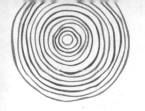

we want to help relieve suffering, either our own or the massive suffering in the world.

Being an energy healer isn't a nine-to-five life. Rather, to be a healer means that your passion for this work is interconnected with all aspects of your life—your personal life and your healing work go hand in hand. The more inner work you do, the higher the planes of consciousness you reach, and the less that will stand in your way while you help those in your world change.

Soon you'll be sending out your higher vibration to the woman silently crying on the subway or calming energy to the manic driver who just cut you off (rather than cursing him!). You don't know these people. They haven't come to you for help. But part of being an energy healer means extending your healing vibration in every direction. Be assured, your vibration will reach them and it will help.

Another point to keep in mind is that healing and curing are not the same thing. Be prepared to discover, as I did, that what we want for someone is not necessarily what Spirit or the person's Higher Self have chosen for that person to experience.

Whether you decide to turn your energy healing into a business or use it only for yourself and your loved ones, I encourage you to keep learning. I know that I am not done learning. I know that as time goes by, I will continue to acquire higher-level skills that I will then share with you. I'm just like you—a work in progress. Every so often, Spirit hands me a new technique. Sometimes it happens when I'm in prayer or meditation. Other times it happens at one of my events while I'm working with a workshop attendee. You never know where or when new gifts will emerge, so always keep your mind open to any messages that come to you. There is always more to learn as you progress in the evolution of consciousness. The deeper you go in meditation and other practices, the more you will become aware of how your unconscious mind works. And the more aware you become, the more opportunity there will be to discard your outdated beliefs and behaviors that are limiting your progress.

When you have finally learned to reach the realms of higher consciousness and spend more and more time communing with your Higher Self, you awaken to your true calling. You will know your purpose in being here on earth in a physical body. You will speak your truth and have compassion for all of human-kind. You will live in the knowledge that no matter what is happening in your life, your authentic self is no further away than your own heart.

You must know by now that you have the potential to do great things. You have the power within you to heal yourself. You have the compassion within to love unconditionally. It's been there all the time. All you have to do is accept and embrace your power and everything it encompasses. This has been the truest purpose of my life as an energy healer: to help you and the millions of people experiencing this global awakening to discover the power to heal and learn how to share that power with the world. Sure, you're going to have moments of doubt, and there will be times when you'll be scared out of your wits, discouraged, disconnected, and under the impression that you're unworthy of such a power. You'll be riddled with all kinds of emotions, both positive and negative. And the untold secret I want you to know is that all healers start out exactly where you are now, yearning for growth, searching for guidance, and determined to change the world. As you continue on what I know will be the spiritual adventure of a lifetime, remember to walk your highest path and always follow your heart. Make compassion and unconditional love your driving force. Only then will you discover your true purpose as the energy healer you are destined to be. Only then will you illuminate the pathway to the glittering sea of opportunity that lies before you. Only then can you truly begin to heal the world.

Go ever forward with an open mind and a hopeful heart, and know with unbending certainty that no matter where your energy healing journey leads, I'll be there to guide you every step along the way.

You have my blessings and my love,

Deborah

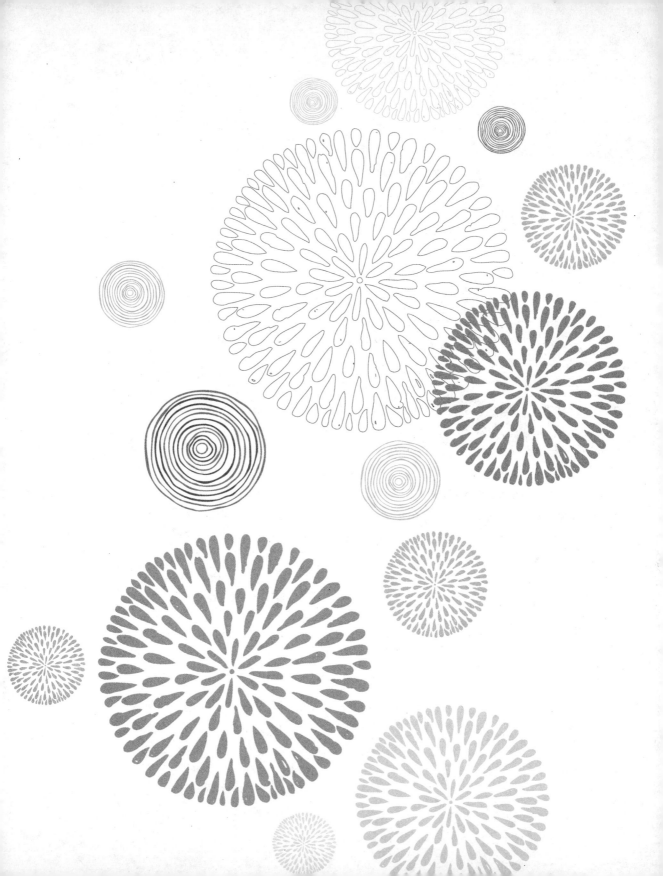

ACKNOWLEDGMENTS

I want to express my real appreciation for all the people whose support took me through the process of this book. It really does take a village!

Many thanks go to my amazing team at Beyond Words Publishing: Richard Cohn, president and publisher, and his lovely wife, Michele, creative director; Lindsay Easterbrooks-Brown, managing editor, who wisely guided me through more revisions than we want to count; Sarah Heilman, developmental editor, whose editorial input was inspirational; Emmalisa Sparrow Wood, production editor, who beautifully tied the whole thing together; and Jackie Hooper, publicist extraordinaire.

Major thanks go to Hannah Hartley, my BFF, marketing genius, tech wizard, talented musician, and all-around totally amazing gal. She has been in and out of my life and it's just not as much fun when she's not part of it.

Big thanks to Parvati Markus for her editorial input and her friendship. I spent over nine months flat on my back with multiple compound fractures of both my leg and arm, and she became my fingers on the keyboard. What a friend! Also super helpful during all the time it took me to get back on my feet was Rita Ribas, part of my support team at home.

I appreciate enormously the efforts of my team and friends at the Deborah King Center. First is Denah Butts, project manager, we couldn't function without her. And no way could we continue to help so many people without my neighbor Tiffany Woodring's magic behind the scenes; what a loyal friend she is. Kathleen Tampoya is another major key to the smooth running of things. And a special thanks to Jan Stake, our accountant, who for more years that I can count has kept everything straight. And I want to mention my dear friend Marilyn Warren for all she has done over the years for me and for the Deborah King Center; she has been here since the very beginning and is now retired.

Last, but never least, is my husband, Eric, who is always at my side. He cheerfully handled the night shifts for nine months of my rehab, and it was only then that I discovered, among his many other accomplishments, that he's a great cook!

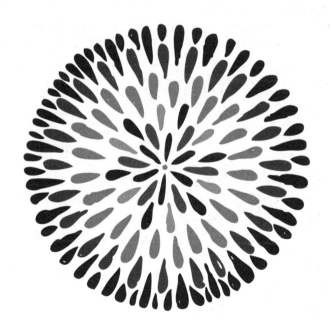

NOTES

Chapter 3: Power Up Your Body

1. Ram Dass, *Miracle of Love: Stories about Neem Karoli Baba* (New Delhi, India: Munshiram Manoharlal Publishers, 1985), 269.
2. Thérèse Tardif, ed., "Saint Padre Pio, the Priest with the Stigmata," *Michael Journal*, May 1, 2002, http://www.michaeljournal.org/stpio.htm.

Chapter 4: The First and Second Chakras

1. Robert Beer, *The Encyclopedia of Tibetan Symbols and Motifs* (Boston: Shambhala Publications, 1999), 142.

Chapter 6: The Fifth and Sixth Chakras

1. David Frawley (Pandit Vamadeva Shastri), "The Flow of Soma," American Institute of Vedic Studies, June 13, 2012, https://vedanet.com/2012/06/13/the-flow-of-soma/.

Chapter 7: The Seventh Chakra, the Soul Star, and Beyond

1. Nancy Red Star, *Star Ancestors: Indian Wisdomkeepers Share the Teachings of the Extraterrestrials* (Rochester, VT: Destiny Books, 2000), 57.

Chapter 8: The Transformative Power of Initiation

1. Joshua David Stone and Gloria Excelsias, "The Seventh Initiation is the Goal of Every Initiate Because It Means Freedom from Rebirth," SelfGrowth.com, August 16, 2011, http://www.selfgrowth.com/articles/the-seventh-initiation-is-the-goal-of-every-initiate-because-it-means-freedom-from-rebirth.

Chapter 10: How to Use Meditation to Heal Yourself

1. Sue McGreevey, "Eight Weeks to a Better Brain," *Harvard Gazette*, January 21, 2011, http://news.harvard.edu/gazette/story/2011/01/eight-weeks-to-a-better-brain/.
2. Angela Eksteins, "Meditation May Be the Future of Anti-Aging, Part I," *Natural News*, February 14, 2010, http://www.naturalnews.com/028157_meditation_longevity.html.

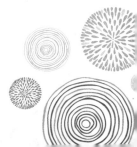

3. Mark Wheeler, "Forever Young: Meditation Might Slow the Age-Related Loss of Gray Matter in the Brain, Say UCLA Researchers," UCLA Newsroom, February 5, 2015, http://newsroom.ucla.edu/releases/forever-young-meditation-might-slow-the-age -related-loss-of-gray-matter-in-the-brain-say-ucla-researchers.

4. Jeanie Lerche Davis, "Meditation Balances the Body's Systems," WebMD, reviewed March 1, 2006, http://www.webmd.com/balance/features/transcendental-meditation.

5. Jo Marchant, "How Meditation Might Ward Off the Effects of Ageing," *The Guardian*, April 23, 2011, http://www.theguardian.com/lifeandstyle/2011/apr/24/meditation -ageing-shamatha-project.

6. Ibid.

Chapter 11: Meet Your Spiritual Guides

1. Paramahansa Yogananda, "Babaji, The Yogi-Christ of Modern India," in *Autobiography of a Yogi*, Yogananda.net, accessed September 5, 2016, http://www.yogananda.net/ay /CHAPTER__33.htm.

Chapter 13: Warding Off Dark Energy

1. Carlos Castaneda, *The Art of Dreaming* (New York: HarperCollins, 1993), 147.

Chapter 15: Your Personal Healing Plan

1. "EWG's 2016 Shopper's Guide to Pesticides in Produce," Environmental Working Group, accessed October 24, 2016, https://www.ewg.org/foodnews/summary.php.

2. Hmwe H. Kyu et al., "Physical Activity and Risk of Breast Cancer, Colon Cancer, Diabetes, Ischemic Heart Disease, and Ischemic Stroke Events: Systematic Review and Dose-Response Meta-Analysis for the Global Burden of Disease Study 2013," *BMJ* 354 (August 9, 2016): 354:i3857.

Chapter 16: Healing with Sound

1. "Kirtan Chanting," Self-Realization Fellowship, accessed September 2016, http://www .yogananda-srf.org/Kirtan_Chanting.aspx#.VwK7OBIrJgg.

2. "The Power of Devotional Chanting, Excerpts from the Writings of Paramahansa Yogananda," Self-Realization Fellowship, accessed September 2016, http://www .yogananda-srf.org/The_Power_of_Devotional_Chanting.aspx#.V60tY5grKhc.

3. Kathleen Barnes, "Music as Medicine: Music Soothes, Energizes and Heals Us," *Natural Awakenings*, accessed September 2016, http://www.naturalawakeningsmag.com /Inspiration-Archive/Music-as-Medicine/.

4. Annaliese and John Stuart Reid, "Ancient Sound Healing," Token Rock, 2011, accessed September 2016, http://www.tokenrock.com/sound_healing/sounds_of_the_ancients .php.

5. "Frequency & the Body," VoiceBio, accessed September 2016, http://www.voicebio.com /freq-and-body.php.

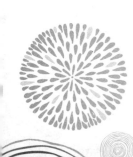

6. "Tuning Forks & Energy Healing," Sound Healing Pathways, accessed September 2016, http://soundhealingpathways.com/sound/tuning-forks/.

7. "Acupuncture with Tuning Forks and Color," Tama-Do Academy, accessed September 2016, http://tama-do.com/roothtmls/acupuncture.html.

8. "Sound Cellular Research," Tama-Do Academy, accessed September 2016, http://tama-do.com/roothtmls/cell-research.html.

9. "Tuning Forks for Sound Therapy," Tools for Wellness, accessed September 2016, http://www.toolsforwellness.com/tuning-forks.html.

10. "Health Benefits: Science View on Health Benefits of Drumming," Drums of Humanity, accessed September 2016, http://drumsofhumanity.org/health-benefits/.

11. B. B. Bittman et al., "Composite Effects of Group Drumming Music Therapy on Modulation of Neuroendocrine-Immune Parameters in Normal Subjects," *Alternative Therapies in Health and Medicine* 7, no. 1 (January 2001): 38–47, http://www.ncbi.nlm.nih.gov/pubmed/11191041.

12. Tom Jacobs, "Music Gets You High," *Salon*, November 23, 2012, http://www.salon.com/2012/11/23/music_gets_you_high/.

Chapter 18: Energy Healing with Your Pets

1. "The Many Meanings of Violet/Purple," Color Wheel Artist, accessed September 2016, http://color-wheel-artist.com/meanings-of-violet.html.

Chapter 19: Share Your Gift of Energy Healing

1. Juan Mascaró, trans., *The Bhagavad Gita* (Baltimore, MD: Penguin Books, 1962), verse 5:12.

Conclusion: Healing Circles

1. Deborah King, *Truth Heals: What You Hide Can Hurt You* (Carlsbad, CA: Hay House, 2009), 2–3.

2. "5 Timeless Truths from the Serenity Prayer That Offer Wisdom in the Modern Age," *The Huffington Post*, March 18, 2014, http://www.huffingtonpost.com/2014/03/18/serenity-prayer-wisdom_n_4965139.html.

3. Printed in the *Indian Opinion, The Collected Works of M. K. Gandhi*, vol. 13 (New Delhi, India, The Publications Division, 1913), 241.

4. Margaret Mitchell and Sidney Howard, *Gone with the Wind*, directed by Victor Fleming (Beverly Hills, CA: Metro-Goldwyn-Mayer [MGM]), DVD.

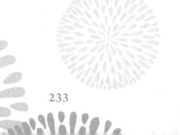

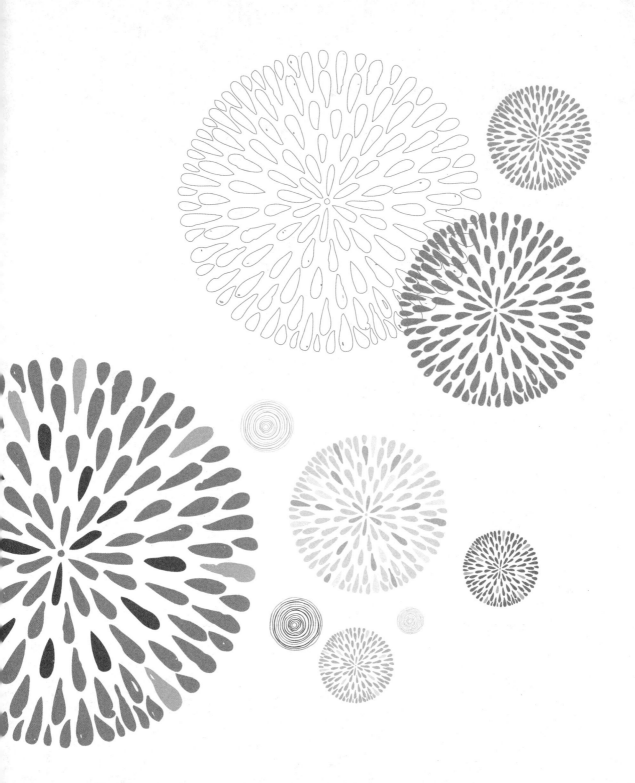

RESOURCES

Deborah King's Website

There are so many wonderful resources available to help you heal, thrive, and grow into the healer you are destined to be. Below you'll find a list of some of the most popular topics and opportunities available through my website, where we can work together via products and online courses. Perhaps we can even meet in person at one of my upcoming events or workshops. No matter where your energy healing journey leads, I hope you know that I'm here to support you, every step along the way.

- To check out my beechwood pendulum, go to: www.deborahking.com/pendulum.

- I teach meditation and provide you with a personalized mantra that is designed just for you at: www.deborahking.com/meditation.

- To see mind/body types in action, go to: www.deborahking.com/mindbody.

- Please add: If you would like to do the Advanced Recapitulation with me, go to: www.deborahking.com/advancedrecapitulation.

- If you're curious to check out the advanced form of meditation I teach that is a sure-fire route to higher initiations, go to: www.deborahking.com/modernmaster.

If you feel a resonance with the Ascended Masters and want to know more about them, I teach an advanced course on this topic. Go to: www.deborahking.com/modernmaster.

To do the Sweeping Breath exercise with me on video, go to: www.deborahking.com/sweeping-breath.

To watch the video where I teach chelation step-by-step, go to: www.deborahking.com/chelation.

If you are curious to learn the LifeForce Energy Healing® technique, I teach it to my Masters-in-Training in my advanced LifeForce Energy Healing® Level IV program. Go to: www.deborahking.com/masters for more information.

You may wish to check out my energy healing school at: www.deborahking.com/school, where you can become certified online and in person.

To join an existing healing circle or to form your own (all at no cost, and we provide everything you'll need to get started!) go to: www.deborahking.com/healing-circle or join me in person in Los Angeles. Find more information at: www.deborahking.com/worldwidehealingday.

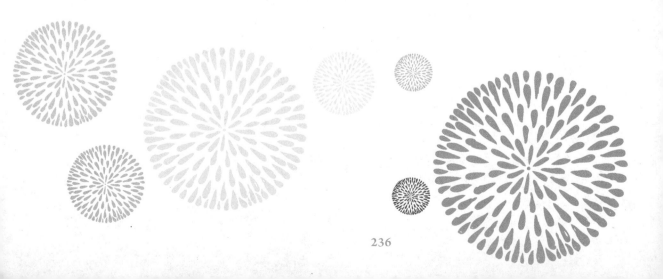

GLOSSARY

affirmations—phrases to repeat to oneself in the practice of positive thinking and self-empowerment to achieve success in anything

ajna—Sanskrit, sixth chakra, the third eye, meaning "to perceive" and "to command"

Akashic **records**—Sanskrit, a library of the thoughts, emotions, and events of all humanity that resides on the etheric plane

amrit—Sanskrit, another word for *soma*, meaning "nectar"

anahata—Sanskrit, the heart chakra

Ascended Masters—enlightened beings who in the past were ordinary humans but who went through a series of initiations into higher levels of consciousness; they are the teachers of ascension

ascension—the process of integrating the light energy of our higher bodies as we rise up in consciousness until we merge in oneness with Source

atma—Sanskrit, the Higher Self in Hindu and Buddhist traditions

atmic—plane of consciousness that identifies with all of life rather than just individual existence

aura—the subtle bodies or levels of the field that surround and interpenetrate the physical body, composed of the etheric, emotional, higher and lower mental, personality, soul, and subtler bodies

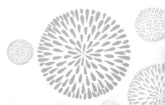

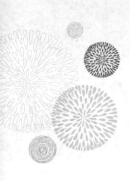

bhavacakra— Sanskrit, a symbolic representation of the cycle of existence, also called the "wheel of life"

bija mantra— Sanskrit, meaning "seed"; a mantra using a one-syllable seed sound to activate chakras

Bindu visarga— Sanskrit, literally meaning "falling of the drop," a point at the back of the head above the sixth chakra and below the seventh chakra

bioplasmic streamers— in Toltec tradition, cobweblike filaments that come out of the "luminous mass" (the human energy field) propelled by emotions

bodhisattva— Sanskrit term in Mahayana Buddhism for a person who can reach nirvana but instead elects to stay on earth out of compassion in order to relieve the suffering of all beings

brachial chakra— the main center of power only in animals that lets you access the animal's whole energy field quickly

Brahma— Hindu deity in charge of creation

Brahman— Sanskrit, the spiritual core of the universe

chakra— Sanskrit for "wheel" or "circle"; the spinning energy centers in, around, and above your body in the form of vortices that receive and send out energy and consciousness

chelation— a hands-on healing technique to clear, charge, and balance the human energy field

Christ light— the vast living presence of totally enlightened consciousness, the love and light that bring about spiritual evolution; everyone has the potential to be "Christed" and to embody love and awareness as did Jesus, who was the most enlightened being in our human history thus far

chromotherapy— light therapy using color to affect mood and health

clairaudience— clear inner hearing beyond normal hearing

clairsentience— clear inner sensing beyond the five physical senses clairvoyance—clear inner sight beyond normal vision

clearing bath—a way to clear slime and negative energy

consciousness—the state or quality of awareness

cords—streamers of light that connect us to each other, chakra to chakra; cords can be positive or negative

core star—the point of light between the third and fourth chakras, connected to the hara line

crystal bowl—a singing bowl made of quartz crystal

dark energy—negative, destructive forces that are harmful to life and evolution

divine intelligence—the intelligence of the universe that we see from the smallest cell to the cosmos

divine plan—the reason we are all here: the purpose of our existence, both collectively and individually, meant for the highest good of all

empowerment—the act of giving an individual the motivation and strength to get healthy, become more conscious, and achieve self-reliance

energy healing—a branch of alternative medicine in which healers use focused intent to attract, conduct, and transmit energy to effect health and well-being

energy vampire—a person who does psychic attacks that drain your energy

esoteric—spiritual knowledge that is hidden and revealed only with entrance into higher levels of consciousness

etheric—the first level of the physical body, which holds the meridians and acupuncture points and also provides the electromagnetic field that surrounds the body

ethics—the moral principles that govern a person's behavior

facilitator—one who can connect to initiatory energy for another

functional channel— the female channel in the Microcosmic Orbit; it runs down the front of the body

Gate of Life— or Door of Life; the small area in the center of the low back at the height of the belly button, a pivot point in Qigong practice

governor channel— the male channel in the Microcosmic Orbit; it starts at the base of the spine and goes up the spine

guru— Sanskrit, the dispeller of darkness

hara line— the line that goes up the spine to the top of the head at a deeper level than the human energy field; connected to life purpose, and exists in the fifth dimension

Higher Self— the aspect of the self that combines the transcendental soul and the Spirit, a reliable source of accurate information

hocokah— Lakota Indian term for a healing circle

human energy field— the field of energy that surrounds and interpenetrates the body, the aura

individuation point— the location three to five feet above your head that connects you to Source

initiation— comes from Latin, meaning "going within"; the shift of perception into higher levels of consciousness

karma— Sanskrit, in Hinduism and Buddhism, the sum of your thoughts, words, and actions in this life and past ones

karmic residue— stored patterns of energy from previous lives

kirtan— Sanskrit, call-and-response chanting

knowings— knowledge consisting of valid information that comes to you from the unified energy field that is available to you once your eighth and higher chakras are open *kundalini*—Sanskrit, meaning "coiling like a snake"; seat of initiatory energy resting at the base of the spine

LifeForce Energy—a combination of energies from the personal energy field and universal energy field

LifeForce Energy Healing™—Deborah King's energy healing technique and the name of her energy healing program

LifeForce Energy Healing Circles™—groups with stated intention for members to heal themselves and others

logoic—the highest level of initiation one can reach while embodied on earth; this is the level of the World Teachers

makara—Sanskrit, the mythological sea creature that carries the seed sound of *Vam*

mandala—Sanskrit, a spiritual symbol, diagram, or geometric pattern that represents the universe

manipura—Sanskrit for the third chakra, meaning "lustrous gem"

mantra—Sanskrit, *man* (mind) and *tra* (liberate); sacred syllable or word that is repeated internally to focus and liberate your mind

Master—an enlightened being who has mastered the ancient wisdom through initiation on the higher planes

meditation—comes from Latin *meditatum*, meaning "to ponder"; a practice that focuses attention inward, calms the mind, and is transformational

Microcosmic Orbit—the circulation-of-light technique from Taoist tradition; used to cultivate and circulate energy

moksha—Sanskrit term for "liberation"

monad—the God Self, connected to the sixth level of initiation

mudra—Sanskrit, a spiritual gesture mostly done with hands and fingers

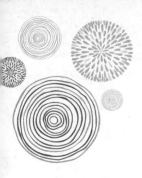

muladhara— Sanskrit for first chakra, meaning "root support"

pendulum— a simple object suspended on a cord that helps locate the chakras and their movement; also used for divination purposes

planes— we exist on seven planes: logoic, monadic, atmic, buddhic, manasic, astral, etheric-physical

prana— Sanskrit, life force, cosmic energy that permeates the universe on all levels; also called **chi** (Chinese) and **qi** (Japanese)

pranic healing— the act of directing your own personal energy toward another person to reinforce their vitality

precognition— knowledge of information about the future

psychic attack— an event that occurs when someone aims their dark or shadow side at you

radiatory healing— a sympathetic resonance between your chakras and someone else's

resonance— vibrations of similar frequency joined together in rhythm

sahaj samadhi— Sanskrit, a master who goes in and out of the highest state of consciousness with each breath

sahasrara— Sanskrit for the seventh chakra, meaning "thousandfold"

samadhi— Sanskrit, absorption in a high state of consciousness

sat-chit-ananda— Sanskrit term for "complete truth, knowledge, and bliss"

seat of the soul— the pineal gland

selfless service— the act of working to relieve suffering but not expecting any personal gain

shakti— Sanskrit, the feminine principle of divine energy

Shen— Chinese, referring to Spirit in traditional Chinese medicine

singing bowl—a type of bowl, either metal or crystal, whose rim vibrates to produce fundamental frequency and several harmonic overtones; used for meditation and sound healing; also called a Tibetan bowl

slimer—a low-level psychic attack that "slimes" you with negative energy

soma—Sanskrit, the nectar of immortality

soul—there is the incarnate soul, the part that is in you for this lifetime, which is a fragment of your transcendental soul: the immortal part of self and the container of all your evolutionary processes

soul star—the eighth chakra

soul seat—the location of purpose and sacred goals, above the heart and over the thymus

Source—the all and everything, both immanent and transcendent; also called Spirit, God, the Divine, the All, etc.

Spirit—the spark of Source in all and everything

spiritual—that which points you toward Soul or Spirit

Stellar Gateway—the passage between the seventh and eighth chakras that lets in divine light and energy so it can flow throughout the body

subconscious—the level of consciousness below normal waking awareness, which holds our accumulation of automatic tendencies

swadhisthana—Sanskrit name for second chakra, meaning "sweetness"

Sweeping Breath—a technique from Toltec shamans to get back energy you left with other people and to return to them their energy that they left in your energy field

tan tien (or **dan tian**)—Chinese, Japanese, area below navel and a third of the way into the body; center of intention and power

telepathic healing— the act of transmitting healing energy to another person's subconscious mind

telepathy— inner communication of thoughts

tingsha— a type of cymbal used in Tibetan Buddhist practices

toning— the act of keeping a sustained single tone using vibrating breath

Tree of Life— also called the "world tree" and the "sacred tree," the Tree of Life is a metaphor in religious and philosophical traditions that represents the connection of all of creation from the underworld to the heavens

tuning forks— instruments for producing sound waves that raise the vibration of an area in the body

unbending intent— concentrated focus on a particular outcome, used by shamans in healing

universal energy field— all the energy in everyone and everything, which permeates the entire universe

uroboros— the image of a serpent biting its tail, forming a complete circle

vectors of force— streams of dark energy aimed at you by another

Vedic tradition— the ancient tradition that shaped Hinduism; its texts, the Vedas, are still used in modern Hinduism

visarga— Sanskrit, a type of breathing sound

vishuddha— Sanskrit term for the fifth chakra, meaning "purification"

vital energy— the life force energy that maintains the health of the body and is also a carrier of consciousness

World Teachers— in the teachings of the Ascended Masters, a World Teacher is an Ascended Master who teaches the ancient wisdom on the world stage, such as Jesus or Buddha

yantra— Sanskrit, a mystical diagram